GET WELL NOW

HEALING YOURSELF WITH FOOD AND THE
POWER OF THE MIND

DR. MEG HAWORTH, PH.D

DELICIOUS AND HEALTHY BOOKS

PRAISE FOR GET WELL NOW

"I love the essential elements about health, food, and body that Dr. Meg is sharing through this book. This will awaken many to a long-awaited freedom with eating and living!"

Dr. Kim D'Eramo, D.O.
Best-Selling Author of *The MindBody Toolkit*
Founder of The American Institute of Mind Body Medicine

"I am convinced that environmental and emotional toxins are the number one cause of disease today. Thankfully, in Get Well Now, Dr. Meg clearly and cleverly lays out a solution - a roadmap anyone can follow - by making simple diet changes, implementing proven mind-body techniques and adopting strategies to reach balance in life!"

Dr. Eric Zielinski, DC
Bestselling author of *The Healing Power of Essential Oils*

"Get Well Now provides a powerful understanding of the toxic effects of the foods we eat, the products we use and the trauma we've suffered. Dr. Meg's practical (and delicious) suggestions are easy enough to implement that anyone who reads this book will experience an expansion in their health consciousness and make lightning-speed progress on their path to total healing."

Tricia Nelson
Best-Selling Author & Founder of *Heal Your Hunger*

"A treasure chest of practical tools to transform the way you eat and think. Dr. Meg Haworth shares the latest research, powerful insights, and her own healing journey to instill the confidence in you that healing is possible, and you can Get Well Now."

Shanna Lee
Author of *The Soul Frequency: Your Healthy, Awakened and Authentic Life* and Founder of TheSoulFrequency.com

"This book provides hope and a different perspective on healing and how powerful the mind can be! The content is extremely valuable and applicable and should be read by anybody who feels frustrated on their health journey or is losing hope. This book provides hope and answers!"

Monica Hershaft, Best-Selling Author of *Treat the Source Not the Symptom, The 3 Pillar System to Get Your Health Back* Motivational Speaker, Health Advocate

Get well Now

Healing Yourself with Food and The Power of The Mind

Copyright 2018 by Meg Haworth, Ph.D

All rights reserved.

Published by Delicious and Healthy Books

Los Angeles, California

GET WELL NOW

HEALING YOURSELF WITH FOOD AND THE POWER OF
THE MIND

Dr. Meg Haworth, Ph.D.

www.meghaworth.com

Delicious and Healthy Books
Los Angeles, California

For all who suffer from a chronic illness –
May you take your healing into your own hands, using food and the
power of your own mind and heart to get well.

And to the memory of Rebecca and Douglass Hayes; cancer took both of
you way too soon. I miss you always and will do all I can to help others
heal in your memory.

And to Chi Ngo Constant; Watching the long slow devastation cancer
wreaked upon your body was heart wrenching. Your brave and valiant
fight was incredibly powerful and inspiring. May the love of our 35-
year friendship enter the hearts of all who read this book, encouraging
them to adopt a life of prevention, healing, tenacity for living life,
emotional and spiritual healing, and self-care.

DISCLAIMER

This book should be read with the understanding that only a medical doctor can diagnose, treat, prescribe medication, prevent, or cure disease by both Federal and State Law. The information in this book is not to be used as a substitute for medical care. You, the reader, are responsible for your health and understand that relying on advice from this book is entirely at your own risk.

ACKNOWLEDGMENTS

I am so grateful to have so many wonderful people in my life who love and support me no matter what new endeavor I pursue. To my wonderful friends and family members who listen to my endless musings about the toxic world we live in, the healing power of food, the sad state of our farming practices, the broken pharmaceutical industry, and contaminated food supply in the U.S., what to eat, what not to eat, how to clear emotions, lose weight, heal ourselves, meditate, and lots of recipe ideas in the process – some things you wanted to hear and many you didn't. To you, I say thank you, with all my heart. You are my people and I love you. To Isabel Maisano, Kathryn, Luis & Rocco Vera, Zach Maisano, Rachel Maisano, Ly Vick Johnson, Kalie Myers, Paul Moore, Debbie Rochlin, Raquel Pacheco, Beth Friedland, Kathleen Bird York, JJ Blair, Claire Burgart, Andy Gerngross, Johanna Watts, Jon Spaihts, Annie Adjchavanich, Chi Constant, and Dr. Kadijah Jones – you are my sacred family of friends and I love you dearly.

For my colleagues in the world of health, wellness, holistic medicine, and natural healing, most especially to JJ Virgin who accepted me into her Mindshare community and helped to lift me up to higher heights. To Dr. Kim D'Eramo, Dr. Peter Kan, Dr. Steven Eisenberg, Chris Wark, Howard Hoffman, Dr. Izabella Wentz, Pedram Shojai, Dr. Stephen Masley, Robyn Openshaw, Joe Cross, Liana Werner Grey, Wynn Claybaugh, Dr. David Friedman, and everyone who has taken time out of your busy schedules to be interviewed on my podcast series. Your wisdom helps the masses transform and your work in the world inspires me every day.

A big thank you to my celebrity chef clients, past and present who helped me become a better chef, menu planner, diet creator, and recipe developer. You have been my laboratory for weight loss, health gain, new recipes and overall health and wellness. Thank you, Michael Weatherly, Dr. Bojana Jankovic Weatherly, Harley Neuman, Daniel Lam, Cote de Pablo, Diego Serrano, Martyn Lawrence Bullard, and Michael Green. A very big thank you to the fabulous Garcia Family, Stephanie, Michael, India, and Elijah, Jill Parker Jones and Gary Tubbs – you gave me my start and took me in like a part of your family. I will always be grateful for your support of my work, the love and the fun times we had together.

For all my clients past and present who have been through spiritual psychotherapy with me, received dietary advice, are part of my private community, are fans of mine, who've asked me questions, listened to my podcasts, sent me messages, sent me books, or who heeded some bit of advice I gave, you are my reason for doing this work. I only hope that I can continue to help you get well and stay well. For all of those who are coming to learn from me, who read this book, or work with me one on one, I am grateful beyond all words.

For my parents, Fred and Dr. Celita Varn, thank you for bringing me into this world, for caring for me and for playing the exact roles you needed to play so I could become who I am today. Mom, thank you for the scientist brain, long medical, sociological, psychological, and health conversations. You inspire me every day. Thank you to Rebecca Hayes for being such an integral part of my life from day one. You were a blessing to our family in every way and you're deeply missed.

For my sisters, Dorothy Grosz, Pauline Brubeck, and Rebecca Pettinelli, thank you for always being there for me and for the love and support you provide for me in the tough times and in the great ones! I love you all! To my niece, Madeleine Krause and nephews, Tom Lamb, Michael Grosz, Greg Grosz, and Charlie Pettinelli, I love you all SO much and hope I can help you and your children live better lives in the generations to come.

A very special thank you to Tom Haworth for all your help and support in the eleventh hour when it was needed most.

Sending so much gratitude and love to my dear friends, Tricia and Roy Nelson for their support, love, and collaborations over the years. You made the final stages of this book and program possible through your intuitive wisdom and unbelievable generosity.

A giant thank you to Shanna Lee and Dr. Eric Zielinski for your insight and brilliance in coaching me to greatness and beyond. You helped me see my blind spots, so I could clarify my vision. Thank you for the love and blessings of your genius. And to Monica Hershaft for endless recommendations for health and wellness and the patience to help me out with some important business assistance.

Many, many thanks to Rita Morales for the book cover design, website design, and for all your digital and technical work. You are the best part of my team!

Thank YOU for reading this book!!! You are brilliant!!!

INTRODUCTION

Life after lightning

It's called out of the blue lightning. A bolt is thrown off from a storm many miles away. It travels across the top of the clouds. It furiously gains energy and speed then suddenly grounds somewhere; where there's no rain and no thunder.

That's what happened to my dear friend and me that July day in 2014, as we sat in the wet sand near the waterline on Venice Beach, California. We were struck, out of the blue, by a bolt of lightning and my life would never, ever be the same.

What does this have to do with you getting well? Everything. You see, when you are diagnosed with a chronic illness from ulcers, to an autoimmune disease to fibromyalgia, to cancer, to suffering a debilitating accident or trauma, you are given an opportunity to begin again. You are delivered into a crucial moment of choice that is tailored specifically for you. What you do in that moment will determine the course of your life . . . or your death.

You have so much more power to get well than you can possibly imagine. You carry within you the wisdom, knowledge, intuitive sense of knowing what's best for you, and even the medicine you need to heal yourself. Your brilliant body is a self-healing machine. What it needs are the proper ingredients to bring about that healing and that creates the process of getting well.

This does not mean it is an easy task. This also does not mean that there is a guarantee that you will make a complete recovery after discovering the healing secrets found in the pages of this book. It means, however, that you have a fighting chance to get well if you have not yet discovered this information. What you do next – the choices you make – contain the power to get you well and keep you there.

I know this. I know this to my core and can say with complete honesty, conviction and certainty that most chronic illnesses can be healed with food and the power of your own mind and heart. How do I know this? Because I have done this myself, not once or twice but *over a dozen times* throughout my 51 years here on planet Earth and, with help, you can too.

I was just 27 when I began to discover the secrets to healing myself. I spent most of the decade prior, in and out of doctor's offices with yet another diagnosis for a different condition. By then I had irritable bowel syndrome, gastritis (a pre-ulcerous condition of the stomach), spastic colon, migraine headaches, post-traumatic stress disorder, chronic depression, vertigo, frequent throat, lung, sinus, and ear infections, ovarian cysts, prolapsed hemorrhoids, and chronic muscle spasms in my neck and upper back from scoliosis and a ruptured disc in my neck. I was a world class mess during a time when I should have been on top of the world. Instead, I spent weeks at a time in bed on a cocktail of pharmaceutical drugs designed to suppress my symptoms, so they could be "managed".

Every doctor I went to said the same thing, these were chronic conditions that I would always have to deal with. Then the doctor would hand me another prescription for a pain killer or antacid medication and tell me to avoid spicy foods. At that point, I was avoiding most foods because nearly everything went right through me. Every place I went; my first thought was to locate the nearest restroom, so I could run to it when the severe abdominal cramping began. It was a horrible way to live and it went on for nearly a decade.

My medicine cabinet was stocked full of all the finest over the counter digestive medications money could buy, none of which worked very well. With each new day, I would have to take all the medicines again and when I ran out, I would go buy more. I used things to keep from having more diarrhea, stop the nausea, dull the throat pain, take after vomiting, quell the constant nausea, calm the fiery hemorrhoids, stop the gas, and keep the acid reflux at bay.

I've now learned that a good gauge of your health is by the drugs in your medicine cabinet. If it is full of everything you need to deal with digestive distress, it's a clear indication that you are eating the wrong foods. Your digestive tract is what determines the overall health of your body, is what I would eventually learn but for that time frame, it was just about getting through the day the best I could.

I would get well from that period in my life. I would become strong after learning how to eat the foods that supported my biology, but I would learn a deeper truth, an unexpected twist to what truly heals the whole person. I would learn the secrets handed down through ancient wisdom by going into my own mind and heart to find the answers I was looking for. I would learn the power of the mind and heart to heal the body and I would discover that true healing happens inside of you and it's done by you.

Ten years later, I thought I had healed everything and decided to fall off the wagon when it came to food and to my own mind and heart. I erroneously thought that my food allergies and sensitivities had "cleared" and I could go back to eating much of the old junk that poisoned me slowly from day one of my life. I thought that because I wasn't running to the bathroom every five minutes that I was strong and healthy, and I could go back to my old ways of eating.

As I did this I started to get sick again. This time new symptoms appeared. They came on gradually and mounted until I realized I had to eliminate what I thought the biggest culprit was, gluten. I did that and felt better. I then used a lot of corn tortilla chips and cheese to fill me up and eventually a whole new host of symptoms appeared.

My hands hurt horribly. I was a celebrity private chef by this point. I would try to open a jar or chop vegetables and I would cry from the pain in my hands. Pain would shoot down my arms and into my fingertips.

I was so fatigued that I felt like I was walking through quicksand each day. I could barely get up the stairs without collapse. I was dropping things without provocation and within a few months I dropped and broke every single glass I owned. My hands would just stop working for no apparent reason. It's as if I had zero control of them.

I would get horrifying pains in my lungs that would make me stop the car and pull over until they passed. I had shortness of breath daily, throughout the day and frequent heart palpitations. Then the vertigo would spin my world each time I laid down. I had overall muscle aches and felt like I had the flu much of the time. I would leave a long day of private chef work in tears as every single part of me hurt.

My friends wondered what happened to me. They rarely saw me because I had no energy for anything other than the work I had to do to support myself in Los Angeles, alone, in one of the most expensive cities in the world. Some days were good, and I never knew when that would happen. I couldn't figure out what was happening, but I knew I had to start investigating.

I called my dear friend, Dr. Kadijah Jones and explained the symptoms to her. She ordered some blood tests and the rule outs began. One test called an Anti-Nuclear Antibodies test, (ANA), showed a positive read for a rare autoimmune disease called Mixed Connective Tissues Disease (MCTD).

I set about the task of researching the western medical approach to this autoimmune disease. The more I read, the worse I felt. I was destined for a life of prednisone, swelling, gnarled hands, and the loss of the use of my muscles, severe pain, and eventual loss of lung and heart capacity. The lung failure is a common side effect of long-term prednisone use, so it was unclear to me whether the disease caused this kind of death or the treatment. It was brutal to think that I would suffer this fate.

I called my family members one by one and shared the sad news. I hated hearing the sadness and fear in their voices. I felt so alone, three thousand miles away from my parents and sisters during this time in my life.

I knew I had to pull myself together and come up with a plan. I had already healed over a dozen illnesses and had extensive training in the power of the mind and the heart to heal the body. I had helped hundreds of other people to heal too. I set out to find someone who had healed MCTD or, at least, had arrested the development of the disease.

The referral to the man who would save my life came from one of my best friends, Kathleen Bird York. She had been seeing an Oriental Medical Doctor herself for a number of years – Dr. Matt Van Benschoten – the most gifted and brilliant healer I ever met whose unconventional diagnostic testing and treatments made all those symptoms disappear with the use of plant-based medicine, environmental changes and diet in about six months.

By the time I went to see the rheumatologist for an official diagnosis for MCTD, Dr. Matt had been treating me for three months. Many of the symptoms had disappeared from my body taking the herbal medicines that were compounded just for me by Dr. Matt. As the rheumatologist examined the blood test reports and examined me, he was incredulous to hear of my improvements, saying I was one of the healthiest patients who had ever come through his office. He did some trigger point tests, told me it must have been a false positive blood test and officially diagnosed me with fibromyalgia with chronic fatigue syndrome. He did a second ANA blood test just to be sure. He had the exact same results as the first, sticking to his opinion of a false positive test . . . twice.

I neither wanted nor needed a diagnosis of MCTD or fibromyalgia. I was happy I was healing the symptoms that had nearly stopped my life with chronic pain, exhaustion and days sleeping for up to fifteen hours straight.

The intense zap of that lightning bolt felt like being hit over the head with a heavy metal object. I watched a plate of white light hit the top of my friend's head and jagged bolts disperse all around us. It was as if we were in one of those static electricity globes where you place your hand on it and watch as the energy arcs towards it. Surreal barely captured the moment.

In our severely disoriented state, when we both acknowledged we had been struck, my friend and I held each other on the beach, crying as we both understood we had just cheated death. In the next moment my friend and I witnessed someone pulling a lifeless man from the surf in front of us. He was large, wearing a wet suit, and probably in his mid-fifties. Our instincts carried both of us, running down the beach towards the guard stand, screaming for help. Before we knew it, the beach was swarmed with emergency vehicles. We knelt in the sand in prayer for this man as we watched the life guard administer CPR to him. I looked up to see the black clouds looming above us and motioned to my friend to leave the beach. I told her we could continue to pray for him from anywhere and we did . . . from Marina Del Rey Hospital. I thank God I had her there with me that day and in the days that would follow as we compared our experiences of healing from that immeasurable voltage.

I passed a paramedic as we were leaving and said, "My friend and I were both struck. We can walk and talk though we are both disoriented, and my head really hurts. Do we need to get checked out?" He looked at me like I had two heads and said, "Yes!!! You've just been struck by lightning and we need to check your heart."

We spent the next six hours in the hospital in Marina Del Rey where they checked our hearts extensively, eventually releasing us out into the world. I had a massive headache that felt like sun burn on the outside of my head and on my brain. It was intense, but I was alive, and I kept telling everyone that I was O.K. though I really wasn't.

In the days that followed, I had an extremely heightened sense of awareness of all my senses, particularly energetically. I could feel a person's pain, sorrow, fears, and instantly understood everyone I knew in a whole different way than I ever had. It was as if I was meeting them all for the first time. And whatever I felt, knew or understood about them, it was ok. I had no judgment, only the peace of understanding them at a deeper level than I had ever been able to before.

My vision was clearer, colors were crisper, the outline around images was sharper and everything had more depth. A person could be standing four feet away and it felt like she was right up against me. A car could drive past me, and it felt like it was slicing through me. A helicopter overhead or a sprinkler outside would go on and it felt like it was going through me. I had been birthed into a whole new reality and I began to go through a life review.

Within a few days, I went to my primary care physician who examined me to find extensive nerve and muscle damage to my legs. I couldn't walk very far without the feeling of collapse and I would have to sit and rest. My memory was terrible, my balance was akin to a drunken sailor, and I had almost no attention span. My usually neat and orderly apartment looked like a bomb had been detonated as I could not concentrate long enough to finish even simple tasks.

My doctor would place me on disability for a month saying she did not want me lifting, standing, or walking for long periods. She had just described my thriving business as a celebrity private chef. I was just about to take on a new client that week and I had to cancel. I had to tell them all that I could not work, and I didn't know how long that would take.

I was given the ultimate time out from the Universe. I was forced to sit down and think about my life and the direction I had been taking. As I did this, one big question kept surfacing; "Am I doing what I really want and living my highest service to humanity?" The immediate answer was, "No."

I had known this for some time. I would be quietly chopping onions in Michael Weatherly's kitchen thinking, "How did I get here? What about my Ph.D. in Transpersonal Psychology? How am I to use that with my knowledge of food and nutrition? I can see how they fit together. How can I show others how they do?" How many veggies I chopped in different celebrity kitchens thinking this thought, I couldn't begin to guess. I just know I had wanted to shift my course for a long time to include a holistic approach to healing with food and the power of the mind and heart. I wanted to share all of it together.

It was in that lightning bolt that this book would eventually find its way into your hands. It was in this time of self-reflection that I would learn to combine my story with my expertise to assist others in healing themselves with food and the powerful mind, body, and soul connection.

No matter how this book finds its way to you, I am thrilled you have the opportunity to learn from my path and life purpose. You can't ever imagine how much.

You are a brilliant being with everything you need to get well and stay well, inside of you and from the Earth around you. That is what this book is about. With all my heart and soul, thank you for reading it.

PART I

FOOD

1

WHAT ARE YOU EATING?

There are upwards of 80,000 chemicals that we are exposed to in the United States today. More than 10,000 of those are in our food supply used as dyes, preservatives, flavorings, emulsifiers, dough conditioners, and sweeteners. These food chemicals are not tested by the FDA, contrary to popular belief. They are tested by the food and chemical companies who make them using research from scientists hired by the companies to conduct these studies. They are often not tested for long term use. We humans are the lab rats for these tests. It can take decades before enough people have died, become ill or are otherwise adversely affected by a particular food chemical before they take it off of the shelves.

A good example of this is hydrogenated oils, also known as trans fats. They were originally used in the 1950's to preserve processed foods and to create margarine as a "healthy" alternative to butter. The process of hydrogenation heats oils to up to two thousand degrees. The result is a plastic like substance that the body does not know how to process, like all of the other food chemicals on the market. The case with hydrogenated oils is that they create free radicals in the body. A free radical is the building block for diseases, particularly cancer, diabetes, and heart disease. It is neither a coincidence nor a surprise that most Americans will die of one or more of those three conditions with the massive levels of hydrogenated oils used to preserve nearly everything in boxes and bags in the grocery store.

It has been known for decades by the natural health community that hydrogenated oils do such massive damage to the body. I remember reading about the dangers of these oils over two decades ago. It took all that time for something to be done about it. Meanwhile, they are still being used and most people have no idea how they are affecting them, especially over time. We place blind faith in food companies who tell us their foods are safe when, by and large, they aren't, not in the slightest. Then we wonder why cancer wards are being filled up with small children to require billions of dollars in treatments and special oncology wings are being added just to house all the children that have to be treated.

You may wonder how something so massive can slip through the cracks. I know I did. It happens when the Food and Drug Administration (FDA) approves something that the food and chemical companies state are "generally recognized as safe", classified as G.R.A.S by the U.S. Government. I don't know about you but "generally safe" is not good enough for my health, for that of the people I love or for anyone else. It is, in large part, due to these laws and lax standards that we are the sickest nation on Earth and other countries that adopt our Western processed and fast food culture are becoming so too.

So, let me break it down for you by exposing the truth on some of the most widely used food chemicals and their basic worst effects, which in the end, result in a slow poisoning of our bodies and a degeneration of health.

Hydrogenated Oils – A method used to keep oils shelf stable, so food products can last for months or even years.

Azodicarbinomide – A chemical dough conditioner used to

preserve bread and make it more light and spongy. It is also used in rubber products. It is so toxic that, in Singapore, if you're caught using it, you can be fined and be sent to prison. It is used in many hotdog and hamburger buns.

Artificial Sweeteners – Chemicals created to sweeten food items like diet sodas, gum, candies, and toothpaste. Shown to eliminate intestinal flora by up to 50%, these chemicals can break down the intestinal tract where nutrients are absorbed into the body, sending toxins into the bloodstream. They have been linked to dizziness, headaches, brain tumors and cancer.

Carageenan – A thickener used in salad dressings, nut & soy milks, ice cream, and jarred sauces to keep them from separating. This food chemical had been heavily linked with bloating, gas, abdominal cramping and colon cancer.

Sodium Nitrites – A preservative used in most cured meats and cold cuts to prevent spoilage and maintain color is strongly linked to colon and stomach cancers.

Food Dyes – Chemical compounds used to enhance the color of a food. Certain dyes have been linked to ADD, ADHD, allergic reactions, severe mood disorders, and cancer.

Glyphosate – The active ingredient in Roundup weed killer, used to spray on conventionally grown produce with known links to cancer.

Mono Sodium Glutamate (MSG) – A chemical flavor enhancer derived from seaweed. MSG is a known excitotoxin that makes brain cells explode and feeds cancer cells. It is hidden under up to 90 different ingredient names. It has been shown to be physically addictive.

The key point is that these food chemicals are being produced to preserve food or to make it look, taste, and smell more appealing so they will sell more. We are more concerned with bottom line profit, convenience, and aesthetically enhanced foods than we are with top of the line health. It is in this backwards way of approaching our most precious collective resource –

the health of our people – that we are stuck in a seemingly
endless loop of chronic diseases.

There's good news though. In fact, it is the very best news a
chronically ill patient can hear. It does not have to be this way!
We ate and thought our way into these illnesses and, in most
cases, we can eat and think our way out of them. It's just knowing
what to eat. But, before we get to that, I think you need to know a
little more . . .

2

QUICK FOOD; SLOW POISON

The more industrialized the society becomes, the more it offers quick solutions for a fast world spinning out of control. In the U.S., there are endless ways to grab a quick bite at a very cheap price. We are duped into the idea that cheaper and faster are better solutions for our lives because they offer ease and fulfill our need to feel filled up and satisfied while tasting great. The truth about that is that we are being controlled by food companies that really aren't producing and supplying real food for us.

The very worst place this way of life is being purveyed is in our families. We are COSTCO'ed, McDonald'ed and Chucky Cheesed to death, quite literally. One of the worst things about this fact is that the majority of those of us who are educated are very aware of the facts, but we somehow disconnect ourselves from the truth as we wolf down the Big Mac and French fries from McDonalds. It is as if we talk ourselves out of the truth and assume that if it is being served and approved by the FDA, that we are safe in some way.

I can't go into a mainstream grocery store anymore without feelings ranging from discomfort to horrified. In the last twenty years, I have learned so much and experienced so much illness due to many of these food products that I can no longer be silent. I feel that by keeping quiet, it would be irresponsible of me. I use those kinds of mainstream grocery stores to buy greeting cards, garbage bags, sponges, and the occasional organic produce item that I think is questionable because they are hopping on a band wagon for sales rather than selling organics because they have a heavy conscience about caring about the health of the people.

The best farms are the small, privately owned farms run by people who care. As organic farming becomes a big industry, I have to wonder what corners the big farms are cutting and what back alley deals are being made in my hometown of Washington D.C. to keep pockets padded, and mouths shut. My nature isn't to be skeptical, in fact, friends have told me over the years that my picture should be next to the word gullible in the dictionary. My nature is to be overly trusting but it is also fundamental that I get to the truth and tell it. It took me many years and tons of study to arrive at the truth of our food supply in the United States. I don't take this lightly and my deepest wish is that you won't either.

The truth is that we are not remotely safe. The average American is slowly dying of food poisoning. It's like the ultimate case of Munchausen's Syndrome brought on by our own government in the approval of some of the worst food chemicals on Earth. Many of these approved chemicals are known carcinogens that are banned by the European Union among other countries worldwide. The thing is, some countries actually care deeply about the health of their people and understand that it lies in our food supply fundamentally. The U.S., being an economically driven society walks a very blurry line between profit and people. In the end, profit usually wins, as evidenced by the overwhelming majority of our city's sky scrapers being occupied by banks.

I say all of this to wake you up and get you to notice what is happening with the most important thing you will do for you and your family all day – feed yourselves. What you eat will determine the course of your life as it will supply the energy to carry out the awesomeness you have to offer the world. You have a responsibility to yourself and to the world to be the BEST you possible. To do that, you will have to feed yourself real, unadulterated food that will make you well and keep you that way. When you consume fast food, you are not accomplishing this end. You are working against yourself in the most fundamental way. You are slowly poisoning yourself and your family.

That may sound extreme to you but if you look more closely at our food industry, it is easy to see that there is little to no nutrition in the food that most us are being fed. As a result, your body is looking for nutrients it needs but it isn't getting so you eat more, and more, and more, only to disappoint your cells that are looking for vitamins, minerals, and whole proteins to survive and thrive.

You can stop this train and get off at the Get Well Now station. It is up to you. I know you can do it. You've got the power and I will supply the know how to make this happen for you. You are powerful beyond measure. I cannot stress this enough and I will keep on reminding you. You have the most incredible power available to you each and every day. You have the power of choice and I am going to help you make lightning power choices that get and keep you well. You deserve this and so does your family.

So, let's look at fast food a little more closely. Think about the fast food chains that they tell us they are healthier, and even salad bars at grocery stores. Are they truly healthy? I say not. Fresh is best but not when it is sprayed with glyphosate, the active ingredient in Roundup weed killer that was finally declared a carcinogen by the World Health Organization in 2016. When chemical fertilizers deplete the soils of their nutrients and pesticides poison the plants, that transfers to us, causing all kinds of havoc in our bodies

The famous scientist, Rachel Carson, released the book Silent Spring in 1964, she warned back then about exactly what is happening now. She told us we are creating a world where cancer is the way most of us will die and that the natural world around us would collapse from the over use of poisons in our environment. This is evidenced by the world bee population dying off from pesticide residue. Do you understand what this means?!?! Bees are what pollinate, otherwise known as, *mate* between the trees. Trees are males or females, just like humans. The bees carry the pollen from the male plant to the female plant to fertilize them since trees can't exactly pursue their mates. Bees do the mating for them. Without the bees, the trees won't produce their fruits, nuts or seeds. Without those, we are sunk as a population of humans that need nourishment from the Earth to survive.

I hope you're understanding the severity of the problem. I do not aim to be an alarmist. But, I do have to tell you that this is ALL so very alarming. We need to do something, and we need to do it fast. Fast food is NOT the answer! Real food is.

So, let's get back to an average dinner at a popular Mexican themed fast food restaurant. Let's say you order two street tacos and a Diet Coke for dinner, one beef and one chicken. You will have a total of four, small corn tortillas with marinated, grilled beef, cilantro, onion and tomato. You can add salsa and guacamole to it as well at the fixings bar. In those two tacos, there is the potential for up to 25 different poisons used in the farming and processing of those foods.

Most of corn in the US is genetically modified. GMO corn is changed at the DNA level, in the seed itself. They used a pesticide called BT toxin in the seed. In addition, they spray the corn crops heavily with Roundup to prevent weeds from growing around the corn. When an insect attempts to eat the mature corn, its stomach explodes. You read that right. So, what is it doing to your stomach?

There was an independent study done on rats. One group was fed GMO corn and the other was fed organic corn. In the group that was fed GMO corn, the majority of the rats became obese, ballooning up to three times their normal size. They also developed malignant tumors all over their bodies. The photographs I saw were so graphic that I couldn't bring myself to share them in my private community on Facebook. I like to educate people but not horrify and disgust them! But, you get the visual. These tumors covered their bodies and stuck out far beyond their normal frames.

Granted they fed these rats a steady diet of GMO corn in huge quantities. But, it took them around nine months to develop tumors and to become obese. The males were 70% more likely to develop cancer and die sooner than the females. So, you may be thinking that you would never consume as much corn as the rats do. But are you aware of how many things you will find GMO corn in? And if you are a regular customer of chain restaurants, thinking it is fresh, healthy fast food, I will have to tell you that this just isn't so.

Next, let's look at the meat served at most restaurants. The beef comes from large scale cattle farms where the use of antibiotics is routine as a preemptive strike to prevent infections and illness. It has been found, however that the antibiotic residue has not only wiped out bacteria that assists in a healthy immune system in the cow, it may have wiped it out in you as well. We have seen the over use of antibiotics create superbugs that no longer respond to other antibiotics. These superbugs have killed many people and will continue as long as we continue this routine use.

We know that what you feed to the animal determines their overall health and well-being. This is particularly evident in zoo animals that are given controlled diets to prevent illness and to keep them strong and healthy while in captivity. The same is true for cattle. They need a specific diet to be healthy too. The farming industry is acutely aware that the cattle are being fed the wrong food that makes them sick, but it gets them fatter faster, so they can turn a profit more quickly. They are being fed GMO corn. If they are what they eat, and we eat them, then we are eating GMO corn, antibiotic residue and the flesh of unhealthy animals fed too much food too fast that is making them sick and us sick in turn. We are what our food eats.

Are you starting to see the trajectory I am on here? What it takes to get your food to the fast food restaurant table or take out bag is multilayered. From the ground up, the produce is sprayed with poison, the animals are fed the wrong food and some of it is even tampered with by scientists who place poison directly into the seed. I could go on with the details of what goes into every ingredient, but I think you're getting the idea. Unless it is organically grown by someone who cares about health and not just profit, it is potentially full of poison and you and your family are swallowing it each and every day.

The more processed the food, the more potential there is for illness in both the short term and the long term. Short term illnesses include headaches, skin rashes, food poisoning, stomach distress, diarrhea, nausea, abdominal cramping, gas, bloating, irritability, depression, congestion, joint pain, weight gain, weight loss, muscle stiffness, lethargy, sneezing, coughing, and any other number of symptoms. If these symptoms are visited over and over again for a long period of time, then long term illnesses like diabetes, cancer, arthritis, thyroiditis and other auto immune diseases can and will likely set in. The reason for this is that processed food lacks the essential vitamins, minerals, and enzymes that are needed to make and keep the body healthy. When you consume a bag of potato chips, for example, you want to keep eating them, not just because they taste good to you but because your body is looking for nutrition every time you take a bite. If your cells are not receiving the proper balance of nutrients, they will ask for more and more food to get what is needed. The problem is that the nutrients never come through most processed foods (foods that come in bags and boxes) so the cells begin to struggle, get sick, mutate and die off. It can take many years of this kind of nutrient starvation before symptoms are felt and then many more before you receive your first chronic illness diagnosis.

I received my first chronic illness diagnosis at the tender age of 23. I was living in Los Angeles for the first time and had only been there for a few months. I was constantly calling in sick to work with nausea, vomiting and chronic sinus infections. I would catch everything that came around and it seemed I was always down for the count with something.

After about a year and a half of chronic sinusitis and digestive problems daily, my doctor said to me; "I think you're allergic to smog. This happens to a lot of new comers to LA." I thought, smog? Allergic to the very air I breathe? Then I took the next round of antibiotics I was prescribed, and everything just kept getting worse and worse until after two and a half years and the LA Riots, I left for the east coast once again.

It would take another four years of suffering and logging hours of sitting in doctor's office waiting rooms only to receive test after test and a snowball effect of diagnoses from gastritis (a pre-ulcerous condition of the stomach), to Irritable Bowel Syndrome, spastic colon, dysthymia (chronic low-grade depression), vertigo, frequent debilitating muscle spasms in my neck and shoulders, and prolapsed hemorrhoids, before I would find any kind of relief and it wasn't in pill form. In fact, the medicine cabinet full of pills wasn't doing any good at all. It would be years before I would learn that pharmaceutical drugs typically manage symptoms but don't actually treat the underlying cause and create true healing. In fact, the underlying cause is never investigated.

The only things I found to create true and lasting healing are food and the power of my own mind and heart. And that is why I wrote this book, to communicate to you that if you have a chronic illness like diabetes, cancer, heart disease, Alzheimer's, dementia, autoimmune diseases, ulcers, IBS, depression, bi-polar disorder, and the list goes on, you have a 70% chance of reversing and completely healing your disease. 70%!!! That is a huge chance of wellness for your life. It worked for me over a dozen times over and I know, with all my heart, that it can work for you too.

Don't wait for getting well soon. Opt to Get Well NOW! In this book, you will learn the basic secrets for wellness and the potential of living a happy life filled with health, the one area we all need to be the wealthiest beings possible.

3

WHAT IS TOXIC BURDEN?

There are more than 80,000 chemicals in the U.S. today. Over 10,000 of them are in our food supply. Those chemicals are produced for one reason, bottom line profits. These chemicals include artificial colors, artificial sweeteners, artificial flavors, preservatives, and additives that make you want to eat more and more of the food because the chemicals in the food you're eating are addictive. Like heroin or cocaine or opiate based pharmaceutical drugs, they are addictive.

Let's take the very popular food flavor enhancer, mono sodium glutamate, MSG. It is an excito-toxin that excites brain cells until they explode. And they don't come back. The feeling you get when you're on this drug is the desire to consume more and more of it. And, it is hidden in most processed food products under up to ninety different ingredient names like autolyzed yeast extract or hydrolyzed vegetable protein. So, when you're eating a bag of nacho cheese Doritos and you can't stop, it's not just the flavor that keeps you munching, it is this chemical that the brain craves more of. The main reason this chemical is used is to keep you buying and consuming the product.

If you go into any Asian grocery store, you will find giant bags of MSG. These bags are clear and filled with a white flaky powder that looks a bit like fake snow. Most Asian restaurants use MSG as a flavor enhancer to keep you eating more and more of their food.

Free glutamic acid is an amino acid that stimulates and over excites not just the brain but also the central nervous system. It has been linked with neurological diseases like ALS (Lou Gehrig's Disease), stroke, Alzheimer's disease, and with numerous symptoms like migraine headaches, dizziness, nausea, vomiting, chest pain, unusual thirst, heart palpitations and conditions like asthma and tachycardia. In addition to these potential side effects and disease states, free glutamates are one of the favorite fuels of cancer cells, feeding them and making tumors grow. We all have cancer cells in our bodies. A healthy immune system just processes them out. Most Americans do not have healthy immune systems due to the lack of nutrition, the high chemical exposure and fueling the fire of cancer cells and tumors with free glutamates and way too much sugar.

Food chemicals like MSG and all their derivatives should be made illegal. They are toxic and create a potential for a cascade of disease states that can slowly poison us. It may have been derived from seaweed in Japan around the time of world war II but there is zero health value in this chemical flavor enhancer.

This is just one chemical that can be contributing to your toxic burden – the amount of chemicals you are exposed to daily in your food and environment. Think about all the chemicals around you in your home right now. You've got cleaning products, laundry detergent, shampoo, lotions, sunscreens, soaps, hair products, make-up, flame retardants on your mattresses and pajamas, scotch guard on your sofa, formaldehyde in your new clothes, fertilizers, herbicides and pesticides sprayed on your lawn and landscaping, chemicals in your water, leaching plastics from water bottles and shrink wrapped meats and produce, air fresheners, perfumes, bug sprays, smog, air pollution, exhaust from cars, off gassing plastics, formaldehyde in your mattress and clothing and the list continues. Also, you're exposed to microwaves, radio waves, cell waves, and wifi that can be disrupting your central nervous system. You are potentially breathing in all of the things I just mentioned, and this doesn't even begin to cover what you are swallowing in your foods and drugs. Can you see the toxic burden around you now?

We live in an incredibly toxic world and it is no wonder that we are the sickest nation on Earth. Of all the toxins in and around you, most of the products in your home and in your food, the ones you use every day contain at least one known carcinogen. The potentially cancer-causing chemicals are known by the food and drug administration as carcinogenic, yet nothing is done to remove these ingredients. Or at least not until enough people have been shown to have died from these poisons through numerous studies and law suits against the corporations that make them.

Everyone seems to think we are safe and that all these chemicals have been approved by the government but as I mentioned before, they sadly are not. In the case of body products, none of them need testing and many of them have been linked to hormone disruption that create autoimmune diseases like Hashimoto's (thyroiditis), and hormone driven cancers. It only takes twenty-six seconds for something you put onto your skin to enter your blood stream. If you're using the same hormone disrupting chemical on your skin every day for many years, it's not too hard to figure out what the problem is. You just need to learn more about these chemicals and what to use instead.

So, what can you do? You can begin to lower your toxic burden by removing these chemicals from your life. The very first thing I suggest you do is to begin within by purchasing organic foods. Glyphosate, the active ingredient in Roundup, an herbicide manufactured by the chemical conglomerate, Monsanto, is used on most conventional produce crops. Glyphosate was declared a carcinogen by the World Health Organization in 2016. This is only one type of poison used in conventional farming. There are hundreds of poisons used on our fruits and vegetables. One apple can have up to 25 different pesticide residues on it because they don't just use one poison, they use a number of them to treat for different bugs, weeds, and fungi. From the soil on up, everything is treated and sprayed to keep as much of the produce sellable as possible.

One friend of mine has a master's degree in agriculture. He said in all of his years of studying farm science, not once did they address the health of the plant for the person consuming it. Every class was based on production and bottom line profit for the farms. I get that we all have to live and pay for our lives, but I don't believe that generating cash should be our top motivation when it comes to food. Our motivation should be how are we going to feed our people to keep them healthy and productive, so they can lead long healthy lives. Are you with me on that?

Another way to lower your toxic burden is to stop eating food chemicals, additives, preservatives, food dyes and chemical sweeteners. You may be thinking, that's all I eat! I am so busy, and I consume everything as I run through my day. I get it. We do this but there are so many ways to get real food in the US that if we all started to make shifts, these food companies that are driven by huge profits with cheap junk that isn't even real food would have to change.

You change. They change. So, start with one thing. Cut back on sodas. Stop putting sweeteners in your coffee and use unsweetened almond milk instead. We have so much sugar and other sweeteners in our foods that our palates don't know how to taste anything real anymore. When you cut out the sweet flavors, you can taste a tomato or spinach, or arugula and these things are full of so much flavor you won't believe it! Your palate will adjust and become more refined when you eat real food, your health will improve, your weight will drop, your mood will shift, and you will heal symptoms you have had for years. Real organic food equals real health.

My mom was an organic gardener. She read Rachel Carson's book Silent Spring in 1964 when it was published. It was the book that changed her life and eventually changed my own. My mom is a scientist, like Rachel Carson was. Carson's book predicted a gloomy future brought on by using so many poisons in our farming practices. She saw the potential of entire eco systems being destroyed and people dying of cancer in droves. She was right. The bees are dying from a particular pesticide and cancer rates are triple what they were in 1964 and are expected to triple again by 2050. If you are a man and you are reading this book, you have a 53% chance of developing cancer. That is massive! Translated, 53 out of 100 men you know will develop cancer. It is an epidemic that we are treating as if it is a normal thing. It's not. It's only "normal" in a chemically smothered society like ours because our usage is way out of control.

Even though mom was an organic gardener and scientist, my dad was the opposite. He loaded the cupboards with junk food. We had Twinkies, Hoho's, Little Debbies, Entenmann's Cheese Danish, powdered doughnuts, frosted flakes (that we added at least two additional teaspoons of sugar to), pop tarts, and dough-nuts from our neighborhood bakery every single Saturday. On Sunday nights we had Chef Boyardee homemade pizzas as we watched The Wonderful World of Disney. To drink, we had Coke, Sprite, and sweet tea with a cup of sugar in every pitcher and we were forced to drink a cup of milk every night with dinner. We didn't eat fast food very often, but we did eat a significant amount of sugar and chemical laden junk. My father now has advanced diabetes. He gives himself a shot on insulin in his belly every single night.

Having two such opposite ways of eating and learning about food was confusing. The sugar laden snacks won hands down. We had no limits on how much we could eat. It was always there for us. We did have to eat our dinner first, but we could always have dessert if we did and we started our days with lots of sugary items.

By the time I reached high school, my lunch most days consisted of Hoho's and milk. I would slowly unroll the Hoho and eat it as I flattened it out, placing the chocolate side on my tongue so it would melt, and I would get that burst of flavor and the sugar rush it provided. On other days I would go with my friends to McDonald's or Tippy's Taco House where I ate lots of cheese and sour cream on greasy ground beef with hard, fried taco shells.

I was constipated all the time during childhood, adolescence and into my adulthood. I would sometimes not have a bowel movement for up to two weeks. I had frequent ear and throat infections, getting strep throat at least once a year. I had frequent bouts with nausea, vomiting and those 24-hour stomach flus that would come through town taking everyone down. I was sick a lot. I went to the doctor a lot. I stayed home from school a lot. I complained of so many symptoms so often that having a ther-mometer in my mouth most days was a common occurrence. Mom was always checking my temperature.

When I look back at what I ate, and how often I was on antibiotics, I can see why I was sick all the time. I mean I can see it now since I've spent most of my adult life studying how to heal myself of multiple illnesses through natural means. I did this, not because I thought it was cool to be different. I did this because it was the only thing that worked.

I think back to my childhood levels of toxic burden and I would say they were high with all the additives, preservatives, sodas, and junk foods we had around the house. Food chemicals were in full swing by the seventies and eighties, preserving every-thing on the supermarket shelves – just like they are today. But, back then, no one knew about the poisons we were consuming. I should say, there were very few conscious people that questioned what we were eating but not nearly to the awareness levels we have now. It's wonderful so many people are aware and not eating processed junk anymore but there is still a very long way to go.

Assessing Your Toxic Burden

As you've been reading this you have probably already been thinking about the things you are exposed to in your current life as well as what you were exposed to as a child in your environment and the foods you consumed. Take a moment and ask yourself the following questions:

1. What did you eat for dinner when you were a child?
2. Were you sick a lot? On antibiotics often?
3. Did you have many of the typical mainstream body products in your home like name brand shampoos like Head and Shoulders, lotions like Vaseline, perfumes, shaving creams, soaps like Dove or Ivory?
4. Were you exposed to radiation from multiple xrays for accidents, medical tests or routine scoliosis screenings?
5. Did you live in an area where they regularly sprayed for mosquitos in the summer time? Or on or near a farm where pesticides, herbicides, fungicides, and chemical fertilizers were used? Or in an industrial area?
6. Did you eat a lot of mainstream food products like Doritos, Twinkies, Chips Ahoy, microwave popcorn, candies like Starburst Fruit Chews and Sour Patch Kids?

7. Did you use bug sprays on your body when you went out in the summertime?
8. Did you ever smoke cigarettes on a regular basis?
9. Did you drink alcoholic beverages at two or more drinks per night, each night or even several times a week?
10. Did you use bug sprays to kill pests in your house or have it professionally treated?
11. Did you eat inexpensive produce that was conventionally farmed and sprayed with pesticides and herbicides thinking that organic was too expensive?
12. Did you eat sandwich meats for lunch most days?
13. Do you eat bacon on a regular basis?
14. Have you eaten conventionally farmed meat products three times a day every day for your whole life?
15. Do you use air fresheners like Glade sprays or plug ins?
16. Do you use mainstream cleaning products like Tide for laundry, 409 for your counter tops, Comet for your bathtubs and sinks, or bleach for clothing or cleaning?
17. Do you have metal amalgam fillings in your teeth?
18. Have you ever used flea dips for your pets?
19. Have you ever been treated for lice?
20. Do you eat bagels, breads, or cereals for breakfast most days?
21. Do you eat readymade pizzas or pasta for dinners often?
22. Do you drink out of plastic water bottles daily?
23. Do you have mostly plastic bowls and plates?
24. Do you heat food in the microwave daily? In plastic containers? With plastic wrap?
25. Do you sleep on a memory foam mattress?
26. Do you have cupboards full of processed foods like

Cheezits, Goldfish crackers, Ritz crackers, Pringles (or other brands) potato chips, and pretzels?
27. Do you have scented candles or plug-ins around your house?
28. Do you use hairsprays, gels, mousse, and detanglers?
29. Do you use makeup brands you get from the drugstore?
30. Do you use nail polish and removers?
31. Are you on one or more pharmaceutical drugs each day?

If you said yes to all of these, your toxic burden is extremely high. If you are living like most mainstream Americans, you have a household much like what these questions describe, and you are in serious need of lowering your toxic burden as soon as possible. Everything on the above list contains poisons that have not been properly tested (except on the American public) and they all have some level of carcinogens in them, placing you in the high-risk category.

If you answered yes to most of these questions, you are still in need of a purge of toxins from your life. If you said yes to only a few of the items, then you are highly educated and proactive, and you can help others with how to live a life with a very low toxic burden. Congratulations to you!

How do I Turn This Around?

The first thing to do is to begin to purchase organic food. You may immediately think you cannot afford that. Most people do so you're not alone there. The truth is that most of us can afford it, we just have to re-work our budgets to do so. Food should be one of your most expensive line items in your budget. Look at where you can take from, so you can give to food. You can cut out cable television, magazine subscriptions, lower your clothing budget, stop eating lunches out, make your own coffee, stop your gym membership and work out at home, wait longer between haircuts, eat dinner at home more, stop impulse purchases, cut memberships you're not using, take less expensive trips closer to home, have a picnic instead of going to a restaurant, have friends over for a potluck, do your own manicures and pedicures. Conscious budgeting saves you tons of money in the long run on paying for a chronic illness that may cause you to lose your job and your life.

Let me give you some perspective here. Cancer rates are astronomical as I shared earlier in this chapter. Cancer care can cost up to $30,000.00 a month. You could go for nine months of treatment. By the end of that, you would have racked up $360,000.00 in chemotherapy and radiation treatments and that doesn't even cover any complications that might arise from the treatment. For most Americans, much of that cost will come out of your pocket. If you bought organic food and kept your immune system strong so cancer would not develop and lowered your toxic burden by getting mainstream body products and cleaning products out of your house, you could live on organics for up to twenty years at that amount of money. That figure doesn't even begin to add up the costs of missed work because the chemo is making you so sick that you can't go.

During and after your cancer treatments, some doctors will tell you to eat organic to help you keep from developing cancer again – but most won't. So now you've got exorbitant medical bills to pay plus now you have to buy organic food?!?! My point is that if you go organic as soon as possible, you could potentially eliminate the mental, emotional, physical and spiritual toll that cancer takes on you, your family, your community, and society.

If you think organic food is expensive, try paying for a chronic illness with loss of work, loss of energy, relationship stress, loss of overall health, prescription drugs, medical tests, over the counter drugs, your precious time, and the emotional toll the whole game of managing your illness takes. Trust me, I have been there and when you can't get out of bed for weeks on end because you are sick from poorly farmed and chemical laden food, body products, and things you are breathing in around you, you lose out big time. Living a life with the lowest toxic burden you can create for you and your family is one of the best gifts you will ever give to yourself and others.

In addition to getting started with eating organic food, you will also want to cut out additives, preservatives, food chemicals, artificial sweeteners and food colorings. These food additives are not well suited to the body because they are not natural substances. Your body doesn't know what to do with them so they either deplete your gut bacteria, as is the case with artificial sweeteners that can cut necessary intestinal flora by up to fifty percent and thus deplete your immune system of proper functioning.

You can begin to lower your toxic burden by cutting out one thing. You might decide to use up the products you have before you purchase the new, organic, clean, products or you may not be able to keep them knowing what you have learned here. The choice is up to you. You are in charge of your health. In our toxic world, you have to be. Your health and wellness are largely up to you. When you make that decision – taking your healing into your own hands – you begin to get well.

4

ARE YOUR BODY PRODUCTS KILLING YOU?

Did you know that body products like lotions, shampoos, makeup, shaving cream, after shave, soaps and deodorants are not regulated? No new laws have been passed in the United States for body products since 1938. Since then, thousands of chemicals have been created to make products do an array of different things from being smooth and creamy to capturing moisture from the air onto your skin. These unknown chemicals have been the subject of much study and debate in recent years as links between them are being made to a number of different chronic diseases that American's are developing and managing with pharmaceutical drugs.

As I mentioned earlier, it takes only 26 seconds for something you put on your skin to enter your blood stream. Once those chemicals get in, they can wreak a ton of havoc on your hormones, immune system and central nervous system.

Certain chemicals are known to be so hazardous to our health that many companies have removed them from their products. You can tell a lot about the toxicity of chemicals from body products by reading labels you find in products and Whole Foods and other health stores by looking at *what is not in the product.*

Here is a short list of popular chemicals you find on the labels of body products that tell you what is not in it:

- Phthalates
- Parabens
- BPA (bisphenyl-a)
- Phosphates
- Fragrance
- Propylene glycol
- Toluene
- Formaldehyde
- Sodium laurel (or laureth) sulfate
- Triclosan

All of these chemicals have been linked to cancer. Many of them are hormone disrupters – meaning they block the proper pathway of your hormones or mimic them, creating a toxic artificial hormone like chemical.

These chemicals take only seconds to get into your bloodstream by way of your skin. Once they do, they can go anywhere in your body. It is theorized that chemicals may collect in your body where the tissue is weakened and where you are placing the most chemicals.

Breast cancer is on the rise. In 97% of breast cancer tumors, they have found high concentrations of parabens, found in most underarm deodorants. The antiperspirant effects of these products stop your sweat glands from naturally producing a natural process of the body.

The lymphatic system of the body is like your personal sewer system. It is meant to help you detoxify and drain toxins out of your body. There are lymph nodes located in groups under your chin, on your neck, in your armpits and at your groin. They collect and drain toxins in the various areas of the body in which they are located. When your body becomes overloaded with toxic foods, body products, and environmental pollution, the lymphatic system can begin to fail, becoming your weak link and potentially developing cancer in the lymphatic system. Body products, particularly deodorants can affect this system adversely.

I have had this odd sixth sense that tells me not to use certain products. As things have come out on the market and gained popularity, I have shied away from the items that I sense are dangerous to health. Among them are sunscreens, anything that says "anti-bacterial", hand sanitizers, and as it turns out, ALL of those items have been linked with the rise in cancer and my gut was correct. If you have a gut feeling not to use a product, then find an alternative solution. There are many.

When choosing body products, I highly recommend using the Environmental Working Group – EWG.org – to help you out. They have lists of products they approve of after very carefully investigating not only the products but the companies that make them. They also have one of my favorite things – a database of chemical ingredients and their level of safety with indicators of links to hormone disruption, autoimmune diseases, and cancer. The organization has high marks for integrity, honesty, and passionate care for human health. Many of my friends who are western medical doctors with a holistic bent recommend EWG. I can't say enough good about all the wonderful things they do to help us all.

5

TURNING YOUR DIET AROUND

W hen I was forced to change that way I ate overnight, it was a hugely daunting task. It was 1995 when my nutritionist lowered the boom on me in terms of my diet. She said I had the worst case of leaky gut syndrome she had ever seen. Basically, my upper intestinal tract was like swiss cheese. She said it was full of holes and was like a toxic free for all. Where nutrition should be absorbed into the body, waste was seeping into my bloodstream, making my body like a landfill of rotting trash. I was thoroughly disgusted but the illnesses all finally made sense to me.

She went on to explain that in 97% of the irritable bowel syndrome cases she saw, if the person ceases to consume gluten and dairy products, the problem goes away. She said there could not even be a little bit of gluten here and there, it had to be total abstinence. I was so far gone and so sick that I had to do something radical or my conditions would have worsened. I believe cancer was up next if I kept eating the way I was eating.

To get an idea of my diet at the time, I was routinely having a bagel with cream cheese for breakfast with a cup of coffee with cream and sugar in it or I would have a Coke in the morning. For lunch, I would have a cheese sandwich with lettuce and tomato with a coke or diet coke. For dinner I would make myself a delicious fettuccini Alfredo with sundried tomatoes and a side salad. I was a vegetarian at the time and derived my protein from mainly milk, cheese, and egg sources. I thought I was being healthy.

For my snacks, I would eat a cup of yogurt or Doritos with Betty Crocker chocolate frosting (I know it sounds gross, but I ended up getting a lot of people hooked on the salty sweetness of this snack). I would often make a yellow cake mix with chocolate frosting or a pan of brownies. Dessert was a Southern tradition and just what you did at the end of a meal. I thought the eggs, the milk, and the flour were healthy items. I thought bread was good for me and butter even better. Milk was a staple item in the refrigerator. I mean what else are you going to have with those brownies to temper the sweetness? I had no earthly idea I was swallowing poison all day long, every single day. None.

When my nutritionist handed me some of her recommended recipes, she said to go to Whole Foods Market where I could find substitutes for the cookies, cakes, and breads I loved so much. She did say, at first, to cut out white sugar. She said my sugars were extremely high and they were contributing greatly to my reoccurring yeast infections. What? Sugar has something to do with yeast infections? Why didn't my doctor tell me that?

She then went on to explain that using antibiotics regularly to fight all the ear, sinus, and throat infections I'd had would deplete my intestines of healthy bacteria. All the sugar I was consuming would then feed the yeast, making it grow and proliferate. My yeast infections were so bad that my eyes, the palms of my hands, the bottoms of my feet, and my breasts would itch. I would also get terrible brain fog and confusion. She also explained that that my diet was also likely connected to my problems with depression.

I could not believe everything she was telling me. How could she hold the keys to this information that was completely opposite of everything that everyone is told to eat? Why didn't my doctor know about the connection between my diet and all of my illnesses? How could my doctor sit by and let me get so sick without addressing the most obvious aspect of living; the nourishment we put into our bodies? I asked her so many questions. She had answers to all of them.

One of the most shocking things I learned was that western medical doctors do not take any nutrition courses! Zero. They are trained mainly in disease states, diagnoses, and pharmaceutical drugs and their uses for treating symptoms; not for healing the underlying cause. Since learning about this, decades ago, I have asked my many medical doctor friends about nutrition education in medical school. All of them concurred that there isn't any – only as food relates to specific conditions like Diabetes or heart disease was nutrition even mentioned.

Western medical doctors don't prescribe healthy diets or herbs because they can't by law. Pharmaceutical companies cannot hold a patent on a whole plant, even if it heals people. They can only isolate the compound of a plant that is reported to do the most good. They then mix that compound with other chemical compounds to make a pharmaceutical drug that can be patented and claimed as the property of the pharmaceutical company that produces the drug. This is one of the reasons why pharmaceutical drugs produce so many side effects; the body does not know what to do with so many foreign chemicals.

They contain chemical compounds, many of which are synthetic, that the body may not process well. If they do contain a plant compound, the other compounds of the plant are discarded. Nature is absolutely brilliant. Plants are made with multiple natural chemical compounds that are meant to have a synergistic effect, meaning they are meant to work together to naturally bring healing to the whole body. Imperfect medicine produces imperfect results.

Death by iatrogenic causes is a term used in western medicine that means; "Induced inadvertently by a physician or surgeon or my medical treatment or diagnostic procedures." According to Merriam Webster dictionary. In the United States alone, there are upwards of 225,000 deaths each year – and that statistic only accounts for hospital related deaths and not those that are caused by pharmaceutical drugs and their side effects. It is the third leading cause of death in the United States. THE THIRD!!! I have to ask the obvious question; if we know that these pharmaceutical drugs, procedures, and mistakes cause so many deaths then how can we continue to call them "inadvertent"? How many people must die of heart attacks from a drug before we take it off the market? How many deaths does it take for patients' families to file a class action law suit? I don't know about you, but I cannot believe that these questions must be asked when it comes to health care.

6

HOW DO I EAT THIS WAY?

At this point, the food companies, restaurants and any other means of providing convenient "food" have trained you to eat a certain way. You grew up on boxed items from mainstream grocery stores and fast food from all the big chains thinking it was all food. It was all safe for your health. Why wouldn't it be? You and everyone you knew were eating the same thing. If you're like me, you're probably in disbelief about the way our society is structured when it comes to food and you especially don't want to believe that the government and the food companies have known all along that their food products can and do make you sick – for some of us we are sick in the short term while for others, it will take years to develop cancer, an autoimmune disease or other chronic illness that you are told just won't go away.

I will never forget the day my nutritionist handed me a few recipes of dishes I had never eaten. She told me to go to Whole Foods Market to get the ingredients and to look for other products there that were gluten free and dairy free. I walked into the store and saw all these tiny boxes of food products that I had never seen before. I became immediately overwhelmed. It was a reality check in my face of all the changes I would have to make in order to get well. I burst into tears and I left the store.

Since that day, I have heard this same story over and over again from clients and friends that had to change their diets overnight to save their health. Making sweeping changes in the arena of your daily eating habits is fundamentally difficult for many reasons that I would discover as I walked the path to eating real food. Eating is one of the most basic experiences we have of bonding to our families, friends and culture at large. When you step outside of tradition and what everyone around you is doing, they begin to feel threatened. They actually take it personally that you are making changes to feel better and they will often begin to make fun of you and single you out because they are uncomfortable with your changes. They will say things that indicate their commitment to eating junk and their discomfort with your commitment not to. You will hear things like; "We all have to die of something." Or; "You have to live life.", "There's no way I am giving up my McDonalds and beer."

These comments will make you feel hurt, isolated and alone. Just know that they are not really directed at you. They are a result of their own fears for their own health. It's their own discomfort being directed back at you. They tend to come from the herd mentality of "this is how things are done" along with the message that food is something to make you feel good emotionally because it tastes so good. This thought is implanted into the culture at large by food companies that are interested in selling their products. They are hypnotizing you with marketing spin that is directed at making greater bottom line profits for their companies. You will see this so clearly as you walk the path towards health.

People will also point out that preservatives benefit you because it keeps food from spoiling, so you won't get sick. It doesn't benefit you. Food companies have trained us to think this way because *it benefits them*. By and large, they are businesses that make your health secondary – or worse – not considered at all. They advertise the pleasure of your palate as being more important than the pleasures of your health and all this marketing has us convinced that "healthy food" will taste bad no matter what you do. This is entirely false. Grappling with the psychological warfare that food companies purvey to gain and maintain huge market shares is one of the aspects of eating well that you will need to overcome to get well.

Another popular belief about food in the US is the idea that eating a healthy diet is more expensive. You are told repeatedly that you will pay so much more for an organic diet than you will for a conventional one. This thought is ingrained in people and it could not be farther from the truth. This is one of the most pervasive and destructive thoughts that prevents most people in our society from getting well and staying well.

So, here are some numbers for you. Cancer care can cost as much as $30,000.00 a month. Over a nine-month course of chemo, radiation and pharmaceutical drugs, you can pay as much as $360,000.00. Much of that sum will come out of your pocket. Any oncologist worth their salt will tell you AFTER YOU HAVE CANCER that you should be eating an organic diet, gluten free, dairy free and sugar free. So now, not only do you have to battle your body being poisoned by chemotherapy drugs that kill many cancer patients, you will also need to buy organic food that you should have been eating in the first place. The doctors wait to tell you after you develop cancer how to prevent it from coming back. But many of them will tell you that you can eat anything you like. Meanwhile, your immune system is being destroyed with poison and you're left with huge bills, changing your diet, and the fight of your life; *for the rest of your life.*

If you begin to eat in a way that significantly reduces or eliminates toxins, clear out environmental toxins by changing your body products, shift your mindset and adopt thinking that can change your life for the better, then you can prevent cancer from happening in many cases. You may be thinking, what if I carry the cancer gene??? This is yet another thought that has seeped into mass consciousness that is completely erroneous. As little as 1-3% of cancer cases are genetic, and, in most cases, those genes can be turned off by your food choices, the life choices you make, and the way you think. The best way to learn about this possibility is to read about the field of epigenetics – the science of changing your genes through your choices.

As you can see, there are some ways of thinking that you will need to conquer to eat well. If you see these thoughts as little speed bumps, good for you! If you see them as giant mountains to climb, put on your hiking boots and get started. It is so worth the climb. You will be amazed at how well you begin to feel in mind, body and soul.

Step One: Create a food plan.

We've all heard the famous quote about failing to plan, right? When you do, you're planning to fail. It's easy to keep on with the same old habits of processed junk and grabbing items off grocery store shelves or ordering in from local restaurants because it's convenient. Adopting a new habit can be daunting at best; even when you know you will benefit from making these changes.

Most of us have lost the connection with our foods. I have talked with hundreds of people that say they either don't like to cook or they simply were never taught how. With a society of food companies and services that do the cooking for you, why would you? To me, this is brought on by the age of fast foods that are cheap and easy to get. The motivation to create a delicious dinner seems to be relegated to the person attempting to impress his or her date or the aspiring chef and at home cook who just happens to like to cook. In losing this fundamental skill as well as the lack of awareness of what is actually in your food, you lose out on one of the most healing and creative moves you can make in your life; preparing your own food.

When you make a connection with your food, it becomes a sensual experience of sight, sound, smell, touch and intuitive insight. Feeling and connecting with your food may sound a bit airy fairy but it's actually quite practical and meaningful. It is the bridge that takes you from being unconscious to being conscious about that most fundamental action you will take all day – nourishing your body with real food. I have found that when clients experience a one on one cooking class with me, along with their menu plans and grocery lists, they have a ton of fun and they discover how incredibly easy feeding yourself healthy food actually is. It isn't daunting. It's fulfilling and when you get the hang of it, it is easy. You will wonder why you didn't do it a whole lot sooner!

When you start your new food plan, I want you to think of it as a lifestyle change. You are adapting to a new way of life, not a temporary fix so you can lose weight for an event or, so you can look good in a swim suit this summer. While those things might be motivators, they aren't long term solutions, especially as you get over the age of forty. While I don't like dropping thoughts like that in your head as we all have different body chemistries, in many people, big changes happen in the body over the age of forty and it becomes a bigger challenge to drop weight and keep it off. Muscle recovery takes longer after a workout, and you see changes in fat deposits, stamina, and skin tone. Having said that, most of that can be halted and reversed through diet and exercise alone, especially if you adopt this kind of diet early in life. Expect to look younger as you focus on real, nutritious food. It is a natural side effect to this way of life. The earlier in your life you can adopt this way of eating, the longer you will look younger.

I started eating like this when I was 27. I had times when I veered of the path by eating gluten and dairy products again and each time I ended up with another diagnosis of a chronic disease that the doctors said could not be healed but I healed it anyway. I did it with food, herbs, meditation, mindset, inner work, exercise and a firm belief that I could and would heal the diagnosis at hand. Everything I just mentioned is necessary to conquering the unconquerable disease that western medicine will tell you is beyond your ability to do so. More about mindset in the second half of this book . . .

When you begin a new food plan, you may shift into foods that you never thought you liked or expected you'd eat. Ever. Growing up, I hated Brussel's sprouts. My mom would serve them, and I would gag on them every single time. They were soggy and bitter, and I absolutely hated them with a passion. I never ate them again until I was nearly forty. I attended a cooking class where the chef prepared fresh Brussels sprouts sautéed in butter and I was in deep, serious, instant love with them. They have been a staple of my diet ever since. It was how they were prepared that made the difference. Mom would purchase frozen Brussel's sprouts. She would boil them, so they were soggy, bitter, and unsavory little cabbage bites that truly made me sick.

Preparation is more than half the battle when it comes to eating truly healthy foods. I personally LOVE flavor and I make sure that all my recipes include that. I mainly use spices from the earth to create flavors in my dishes. Most people add cream and cheese to make things taste richer and more delicious. But, if you want to reduce inflammation then learning how to use spices from the Earth and how to balance them not only adds flavor but they have compounds that heal conditions in the body while making your palate happy too. Here are just a few of them:

Cinnamon – Stabilizes blood sugar. Great in meat dishes with chili powder, cayenne pepper, sea salt, and garlic powder.

Cayenne Pepper – Improves blood circulation. Excellent added to vegetable sautés, soups, smoothies and pancakes. The spice brings out the sweet. Cayenne loves most spice mixtures.

Oregano – Has antibacterial and antimicrobial properties

(particularly in oil form). This spice is excellent in soups, tomato sauces, on sweet potatoes, on eggs, and in salads.

Curry Powder – Has anti-cancer, digestive and anti-inflammatory properties. This is wonderful with meats and vegetables alike. Combine curry powder with cumin, turmeric, sea salt, garlic powder, and cayenne pepper for an incredible combination of flavor and health value.

Turmeric – Anti-cancer, antioxidant, anti-inflammatory, and improves brain function.

Garlic – Anti-bacterial, anti-microbial, and anti-fungal properties (especially when consumed raw). Infections have been killed using garlic alone. Use in pesto, roasted red pepper sauces, guacamole, tuna salad, salad dressings, and add a pressed clove or two to organic tomato sauces at the last minute for extra flavor and health value.

Sea Salt – High mineral content. Excellent in anything from cookies, smoothies, soups, eggs, meats, and vegetables. It is the one spice I use in everything. Salt is needed for every system of the body to function. High blood pressure or not, it is necessary to life. My blood pressure is very low, so my doctor advised salting everything. Celtic, Himalayan, and Black Lava salts are the highest in mineral content.

Those are just a few of my favorite spices and most used spices. When I create a dish, I think about flavor, nutrition, enjoyment, aroma, and happiness. Food is perhaps the greatest healing force we have available to us. Spice it up to bring your system into happy balance and joyful appreciation of the wonderful food you're about to eat!

Planning for Eating

As a celebrity private chef, I have been crafting food plans specific to the needs of my famous clients for over a decade. Prior to that, I owned a Bed & Breakfast and retreat center in South

Carolina where I cooked dishes made from the organic garden for guests and taught cooking classes at Earth Fare natural market in Columbia. I have had a lot of experience with creating dishes out of few ingredients, living way out in the country, shopping at markets in the back woods of the deep South. I also learned how to eat around a population of people that were more concerned with tradition when it comes to eating than with health. I used to joke that they fried everything in the south except the coleslaw and I am sure someone has tried!

That is not to say they're wrong for eating the way they do. I used to eat the exact same way. I was raised by southern parents on sweet tea, biscuits, cakes, cookies and foods smothered in gravy too. I have learned that in the times we are, food quality is where we need to focus our attention if we want to get well and stay that way. I don't believe we necessarily have to eliminate everything we love. We just may have to swap out some items for our wellness. I still make a mean meatloaf. I just do it with organic ingredients. Basically, they're ingredients my grandmother used to cook with because, back then, they were just ingredients. Now, they are mainly sprayed with poisons, genetically altered, or have potentially toxic packaging. I want to help you get the poison out of your diet, so you can get to feeling better.

Sample Food Plan

Below is a menu plan I created for one of my celebrity clients. His goal was to lose twenty pounds and to maintain his weight for his incredibly busy schedule of filming for television, press, and media for his hit show.

Day 1:

B – Two Scrambled Eggs with ½ an Avocado & Tomato

L – Rosemary Chicken Salad with fresh Spinach, Carrots, Tomato, Cucumber, Cranberries and Almonds

D – Turkey Meatloaf with Roasted Broccoli and roasted sweet potato

Day 2:

B – Dr. Meg's Zero Sugar Morning Smoothie

L – Turkey Burgers with Roasted Red Pepper Sauce, Arugula Cucumber Tomato, Cranberries, Carrots and Pecans

D – Chicken Marsala with Garlic Green Beans and Roasted Butternut Squash

Day 3:

B – Mini Vegetable Frittatas

L – Minestrone Soup with Side Salad

D – Turkey Meatloaf with Roasted Broccoli

Day 4:

B – Dr. Meg's Zero Sugar Morning Smoothie

L – Herbs de Provence Chicken Salad with fresh Spinach, Carrots, Tomato, Cucumber, Cranberries and Pecans

D – Grilled Top Sirloin Steak with Roasted Cauliflower and Carrots and Sautéed Spinach

Day 5:

B - Mini Vegetable Frittatas

L – Minestrone Soup with Side Salad

D – Chicken Marsala with Garlic Green Beans and Roasted Butternut Squash & Pecans

For you, this menu may be daunting. It is a lot of different dishes that would take me at least five hours to prepare, package and clean up after 1.5 hours of grocery shopping (at two different stores) plus menu planning time and approval from the client. Most people not only don't have the time to do the work of a celebrity chef, but they also don't have the level of skill required to execute a menu of this nature on a weekly basis. I wanted to show you this to give you an idea of what my celebrity clients eat as well as how planning can go for menus for you in your daily life.

As you can see, I have repeated two of the dinners twice. This is due to the size and time it takes to make one dish. I try to make the preparation easier on myself when I have a day full of work like this, so I will go to Trader Joe's and purchase as much organic, prepackaged produce as I can. They have bags of greens like spinach, kale and mixed baby greens for very small amounts of money. Spinach is only $1.99 a bag and one bag can make you three salads or two sides of sautéed spinach with garlic and onion.

In addition to two repeat dinner dishes over four nights, I have what I think of as the one-off dinner. In this case, it's the one night he will get a 4-6-ounce portion of red meat for iron, protein, and b vitamins. I think about several factors when I create a menu plan for a client from likes and dislikes to nutrition, enjoyment, satiation, and even the weather (which I check first). I find that most people don't want chili in the summer. They want dinner salads with warm, hearty food in the winter time.

For your purposes, you may want to do super simple things for your menu plan. Say you're cooking for two people, three meals a day for a five-day work week. This process will go very fast if both of you pitch in and talk about menu, plan your grocery lists, shop together, and cook and clean together. The whole process from start to finish may only take you about three or four hours. It's a bonding experience that can allow you to spend time together that you wouldn't normally.

If you do it this way, consider the following menu plan made for two people:

Menu Plan II:
4 Pan Seared Salmon
6 Grilled Chicken

4 Organic Hamburgers

1 Container Dairy Free Lemon Mint Pistachio Pesto

1 Container of Navy Beans with Roma Tomatoes & Avocado with Lemon Juice, Sea Salt and Pepper

1 Container Roasted Brussel's Sprouts

1 Container Quinoa with Apricots and Walnuts

This is a super simple plan.

You have the container in the refrigerator and all you have to do is put a plate together based on what you feel like having. This plan will take you about 1.5 hours to prepare.

When you have a plan like this, keep things on hand like a bag of organic arugula, avocados, fresh lemons, cherry tomatoes, cucumbers, carrots, celery, pecans, almonds, hemp seeds, sunflower seeds and extra virgin olive oil. You can add any of these items to your plate.

For instance, I would place arugula on the bottom of my plate. I would put the quinoa dish on top of that, add a piece of salmon with pesto and be eating like a queen!

For another dinner that week, I would have a side salad of arugula with the navy bean salad on top with roasted Brussels sprouts, pecans and grilled chicken topped with avocado. I would then add hot sauce to the mix to spice it up, speed metabolism and improve blood circulation.

A simple plan like this makes eating this way easy, creative, enjoyable and you've got fast food sitting in your refrigerator that you don't have to do very much to in order to have great meals all week long. For breakfast, you can make my zero-sugar chocolate green smoothie or scrambled pasture raised eggs with avocado and hot sauce. You eat a diet like this and you will be feeling amazing in no time flat AND, you will be eating real, delicious, super simple meals that make your heart sing and your bank account will be fuller because you're not purchasing impulse items because you waited until you were too hungry to go to the store and would literally eat anything. You then grab poorly farmed food that's full of poisonous residues, hormones, and animals fed the worst possible diets for their own health, let alone yours.

Sourcing Ingredients

Most people think that an organic diet of whole, real food will be way too expensive for the average family to afford. The truth is that you can do the food plans I have shared with you for around $100.00 a week. Shopping at stores like Trader Joe's for produce and organic meats and wild caught fish is perhaps the best way I know to keep your costs down.

I prefer Whole Foods Market for meats and fish because of their strict standards on where they source their ingredients. They have people in the company called foragers who go to the farms and inspect them on a regular basis to build and maintain relationships with the farmers and to continue watching their compliance with company standards. Whole Foods is particularly my number one choice for their seafood standards. Their seafood teams receive ongoing training on where seafood is sourced, and they maintain close relations with The Marine Stewardship Council – https://www.msc.org/ - an international non-profit organization that certifies fisheries and businesses around the world for high standards on wild capture fishing. When you shop for fish, ask if they were MSC certified.

Trader Joe's is rolling out a new store that will help consumers get organic and fresh produce at deeply discounted prices. Whole Foods Market has already opened their flagship store called 365 in the Silverlake area of Los Angeles. Their in-house brand, 365 has been offering hundreds of organic products in their stores for many years at competitive prices that are designed to save you money at checkout. Most mainstream grocery stores now have organic food sections in their produce departments as well as in the center aisles for everything from cereal to ketchup. It's a way to keep costs down for them and for shoppers without sacrificing quality.

There are multiple services that now deliver organic produce right to your door each week. You will have to learn to be creative in the kitchen with most services like this because you will get what is being harvested that week. They typically have you choose vegetables and fruits in combination or just one or the other.

There are also other services that deliver frozen organic meats and or produce all year round for you. When I owned a Bed & Breakfast and Healing Retreat Center in South Carolina in the early two thousands, I had one of these services. I lived fifty miles from the nearest city and organic produce was not available at all at the local Piggly Wiggly, Food Lion or Wal-Mart Super Center. We also had a huge organic garden that we routinely cooked from. We would even forage from the land around us for wild greens and dandelions.

One of my favorite memories at the B&B was when dear friends of ours came down from DC, where my then husband and I are from, and stayed with us for a long weekend. We went out to the garden and picked a couple of pumpkins. We made pumpkin soup and pie and it was some of the best food I have ever eaten. There is nothing more brilliant than fresh food cooked out of your own garden and shared with friends and family. If you can't garden, and you live far away from any place with real organic food, these frozen organic services are fantastic.

Another absolutely wonderful service that I highly recommend is an online organic, whole food, grocery store called Thrive Market. It's like Costco meets Whole Foods with online delivery anywhere you are. You can get body products, supplements, food, cleaning products, nuts, snacks, and just about everything you can get at a natural food store at deep discounts.

You only need to purchase a membership. When you do purchase your membership, Thrive Market donates it to a low-income family so that organic food and products can also be accessible to them. Their social mission is brilliant and they are constantly offering free products and big sales. To join up, use this link: www.meghaworth.com/thrive-market. It's the best place to purchase the ingredients for my protein powder too – raw cacao powder, hemp powder, maca powder, chia seeds, stevia, cinnamon, cayenne pepper, and golden flax seeds.

With the availability of organic produce going up along with the demand for it, we will have many more resources like the ones I mentioned above in the years to come. You do vote with your dollars when you choose organic. It may be a stretch financially at first but the long-term gain in health is indisputable. As a single entrepreneur living alone in one of the most expensive cities in the world, Los Angeles, my income is always going up and down. In the down times, I move my budget around, so I will always be able to eat organic food. I cancel subscriptions, color my own hair and wait longer between haircuts, do my own pedicures, cancel magazine subscriptions, stop purchasing clothing (or go to thrift stores if I really need something), cut out movies, dinners out, or whatever it takes so I can eat good clean food. Having been so sick with over a dozen illnesses, then gaining my health back better than it ever was before is enough motivation for me to stay the course with real, clean, delicious, nutritious, organic food. I encourage you to do the same for you and your family. It's much easier than you may think!

Step two: Implement the food plan.

For most people that choose to or *need to* eat this way, you will want to go with the second food plan in which you make several dishes a week and have items on hand to mix and match different meals with. This type of plan is incredibly easy and can be done over the course of a few short hours on a Sunday afternoon or evening.

Once you write down what you want to make for that week, the next step is to make the grocery list. My menu and lists for my celebrity private chef clients look like this:

MENU:
4 Pan Seared Salmon
6 Grilled Chicken
4 Organic Hamburgers
1 Small Container Dairy Free Lemon Mint Pistachio Pesto
1 Medium Container of Navy Beans with Roma Tomatoes & Avocado with Lemon Juice, Sea Salt and Pepper
1 Large Container Roasted Brussel's Sprouts
1 Large Container Quinoa with Apricots and Walnuts

Trader Joe'sWhole Foods Market
Produce:Produce:
1 bag arugula3 Roma tomatoes
4 avocadosBulk:
1 box fresh basil10 dried apricots
1 small box mint **Boxed or Bottled:**
4 prepared Brussel's Sprouts2 cans of navy beans
Fresh garlicSeafood/Meat:
2 lemons4 wild caught salmon 6-7
Boxed or bottled:ounces each
1 bag quinoa3 organic chicken
1 box organic chicken brothbreasts 8 oz. halved

Meat:
1 package organic hamburger (or Bison)

*The people at the meat and seafood counter at Whole Foods Markets will butterfly and slice chicken breasts in half so you have about 4-ounce pieces at a serving. If you're working out a lot, you will want to eat the whole 8 oz. piece. Americans focus too much on meats and not enough on vegetables. Always make vegetables the main event on your plate and have at least one vegan day each week (no animal proteins).

Items that are typically on Hand in the kitchen:
Sea Salt (I like Trader Joe's Pink Himalayan in the grinder).
Black pepper (also in a grinder)
Garlic Powder (I like Trader Joe's brand)
Walnuts (TJ's)
Pistachio nut meats (TJ's)
Extra Virgin Olive Oil (Whole Foods 365 Organic brand)

Snacks:
Organic Hummus (Trader Joe's) with organic carrot sticks
Baba ganoush with cucumber rounds (Trader Joe's)
Kale Chips (either homemade or Trader Joe's)
Olive tapenade with gluten free rice crackers (Trader Joe's)
When you have things like hummus and olive tapenade on hand, you can put those things on chicken and fish and on salads. The two together, taste delicious!

Desserts:
Mixed organic berries with almond milk and cinnamon
Raw Chocolate Pudding (vegan)
Spicy Raw Coconut Cacao Balls
Dr. Megs Raw Chocolate Smoothie (pour some in a bowl with pecans, berries, coconut, almond butter and sea salt for a deli-

cious snack or just have it by itself. I make a pitcher at a time and have it on hand for two or three days for breakfasts and snacks). For all of the recipes in this food plan, go to my blog at www.meghaworth.com/blog and type the name in the search field. Many of them are made into videos for you with lots of extra suggestions.

As you can see, the grocery lists for these recipes are not long at all. If you have the seasoning ingredients and nuts on hand in the kitchen already, you should pay around $100 for two people for these items from these stores for the week. This doesn't include breakfasts and snacks. If you make smoothies for breakfast and have real food snacks on hand, you may pay about $25.00 more per week on average. Your main beverage will be water every day throughout the day. Sparkling mineral waters like Pellegrino or Gerolsteiner with fresh lemon or lime are also great drinks to have on hand.

Tools for the Kitchen

The kinds of cookware and the kitchen accessories you use are critical to having a great outcome for your food. This is true for both health and ease of cooking. Some cookware (most non-stick) has been linked to cancer and autoimmune diseases. I highly recommend using stainless steel, glass, and/or enamel coated cast iron cookware.

There are all kinds of ways to get superior cookware at a fraction of the cost. Here are some:

E-Bay

Yard or estate sales

Thrift stores like Goodwill or Salvation Army

Bed Bath & Beyond 20% discount coupons

Marshall's TJ Maxx or other discount stores

Kitchen discount supply stores

As for knives. You can simply go to a place like Marshall's and get excellent deals on knives. Get something that has some weight to it. The weight of the knife helps you cut into things more quickly and easily. Check to see if the knife was forged or stamped. Forged means it was individually made by a knife smith. Stamped is machine made and typically of lower quality. A good sharp knife will make the biggest difference in the kitchen. Use a Chef's Knife or Santoku Knife for best results. A dull knife can make anyone not want to cook as it is very frustrating.

Here are the materials you will need to carry out a food plan like the one above:

High Speed Blender like a Blendtec or Vitamix

Food Processor

Wooden Cutting Board

Sharp Chef's Knife

Soup Pot

Skillet

A Vegetable Spiralizer (if you want to make zucchini noodles)

Food storage containers (glass is best or BPA free plastic)

There are so many ways to cook your own food. You can hire someone right out of culinary school for only $15.00 - $20.00 an hour. It should take 5-6 hours or less to cook a list of food like the above. That includes clean up and shopping. That's $75.00 a week plus groceries. Everything you've got will be used (unlike when you over buy thinking you'll use something, only to watch it end up in the trash.)

That is only around $75.00 a week for one day of cooking. It's a bargain! You will spend so much more than that at restaurants and the food will not be good for you in most instances. It will likely be pesticide laden conventional produce with poorly farmed meats, and food chemicals, with excess sodium and sugar.

I have chef clients who were embarrassed that they had hired me. They didn't want friends to know at first because they felt like it was something only rich people did. They couldn't even call me a chef in the beginning. They called me the "cooker lady". They did that because they had grown up thinking this was a luxury. They both had their own businesses and worked beyond full time, so my help ended up being a necessity, not a luxury. They needed me to help them with food that wouldn't make them gain weight. They used to get prepared foods at the deli counter in nice stores that was supposed to be healthy. The problem was it was making them fat and sick from added sugar, industrial seed oils, and preservatives. Having me solved that problem for them.

When they hired me, they began to see (as the weight dropped off) that it was one of the best decisions they made. They even came to see me as one of their strongest assets because I took care of not only their waistlines while providing food they loved, I took care of their health. Years later, they would proudly speak of the amazing chef that keeps them thin and happy.

This could be you. You just have to shift your mindset and think differently about how you get fed, how you get healthy and how nourishment comes to you. You may find that when you do the math for both now and later in the prevention of chronic illnesses, you have saved not only hundreds of thousands of dollars, you have saved your life.

I did the math earlier in this book as to what a chronic illness like cancer or an autoimmune disease can cost you. It is far, far, more expensive than you can imagine. Your life will become about managing your health and paying for all the various treatments you need, missing work, going on disability, missing out on events with your family and friends, basing everything you do on how you are feeling that day is horribly exhausting. It is difficult, and it makes you feel depressed, damaged, and alone. If you can prevent that, wouldn't you want to at least give it a shot for six months or so to see how you do?

I am not saying that you can reverse or prevent all illness. This book wasn't written to diagnose or treat your conditions. I am saying that there is overwhelming evidence that shows time and time again that eating certain foods while avoiding others can help reverse the disease process and make you well. I have seen this happen with my own body and with my clients, colleagues, and friends who have adopted this kind of diet and lifestyle. Isn't that worth trying for?

Step Three: What to Eat in a Restaurant.

If you want to truly eat a diet of real, whole, organic, food, I recommend not eating in restaurants very often at all. If you do, the very best ones are the privately-owned restaurants where you can build a relationship with the chef. Many of these chefs are very aware of quality and source the ingredients themselves from connections they have made and nurtured for many years. These chefs care about food quality and who they do business with. You may pay a little more to dine at these restaurants, but it is worth every penny.

In privately owned restaurants, they are typically accommodating when it comes to giving their customers what they want, like and need. If you see an ingredient listed in one of the dishes on the menu, that means it is back in the kitchen, so you can effectively create a plate full of the food that you want prepared with extra virgin olive oil rather than butter or steamed, grilled, or however you like your food.

I recognize that when you travel to certain parts of the country, you will not be able to find these kinds of restaurants. You may end up in one of the big chain places where everyone eats at their own risk. Soups and many other dishes in these restaurants are premade and trucked in from other locations in plastic bags containing toxic chemicals that cause cancer, weight gain, diabetes, autoimmune diseases and all hormone related disorders. The plastic bags and containers are the least of it. That food was originally farmed using poisons, hormones, antibiotics from animals being fed the absolute wrong diet for the animal you are consuming. Often, the animal that you are eating was sick at the time it was slaughtered – *because it was eating the wrong diet*. That translates to your body and your level of health. You are what your food eats.

Unless it says certified organic, it is poison in the US and that is the sad truth. We can change this with our dollars by making different choices. This change is in process and I ask you with all my heart and soul to become a part of this change. It is up to all of us to do it.

If you do find yourself in a big chain restaurant, stick to dishes that focus on meats and vegetables. A grilled piece of fish or steak with a side of broccoli and a baked potato with Italian dressing on it is probably the best choice you can make. They also have salad bars at these places typically. While that comes with another set of issues because of the preservatives they spray on the vegetables to keep them crisp and fresh can cause food reactions and illness, at least there's something fresh available.

When I was 27 or 28 I went on a trip with girlfriends to the eastern shore of Delaware for a weekend. I had already cut out gluten, dairy, sugar, fried foods, corn, peanuts, citrus, alcohol and caffeine to save my health. I was feeling tons better and had lost twenty-five pounds cutting out the offending foods.

We stopped at a big chain restaurant on the way home for lunch. Some of my friends really wanted ice cream sundaes. I just wanted some meat and vegetables because I knew they would make me feel good for the ride home. The only thing I could eat was on the senior menu. It was steamed broccoli, a baked potato and a ribeye steak. I ordered it and was told by the waitress that I couldn't order from the senior menu. I explained that I had food allergies and anything else on the menu would make me sick. She continued to argue that the senior plates were also discounted to help senior citizens. I told her to charge me extra then. Whatever it took so I could order the food that I knew I could eat without doubling over in pain, running to the restroom, being nauseous for days, developing a migraine or an infection. She finally relented and brought me this menu item. Arguing with her about my food allergies was surreal. It's as if she didn't believe me and didn't want to.

It struck me at that time that this is what we do in America. We eat ice cream, cakes, candies, processed junk, poorly farmed meats, overly rich foods, fried anything, and avoid vegetables until we become sick. Apparently, most seniors have to change their diets to real, whole foods because they've finally broken down their digestive tracts to the point of no return. For me, it only took until I was about twenty for the symptoms to become so loud that I started the rounds of doctor's office waiting rooms for diagnoses and drugs that never helped to treat the underlying cause. Food helped. Food healed, and my mind and spirit did the rest.

Another alternative to restaurants when you're traveling is to find a Whole Foods Market (or other natural foods store) and purchase prepared foods or buy organic produce. You can eat a bag of mixed greens just like you would a bag of potato chips. Carry flatware in your car and get an avocado. You can halve it with your knife and scoop it out with your spoon and eat it. Have an orange, pear, plum, or apple for something sweet. Carry almonds or other nuts with you to have healthy fats on hand for you to snack on. Drink plenty of water to help you process out waste and to fill you up if you get hungry while out and about.

This new way of eating requires a mindset that asks you to plan ahead so you will stay fed, hydrated, and healthy. You will have to become aware of taking care of yourself and include it as a top priority that will become as natural as brushing your teeth or putting on your clothes each morning. You can make this a simple habit that you expect to do each day.

Step Four: What to eat at parties and events.

I am very lucky to live in California. When I go to a potluck, people bring salads, quinoa dishes, grilled or roasted vegetables, and all manner of gluten and dairy free, real food items. This is often the case but not always. Many parties I go to have vegetables to eat but even I don't always want those. What I usually do before I go to a party or an event is I eat a nice big lunch or dinner prepared by me. This way I go to the party full and don't feel tempted to eat things that I know will make me sick or feel bad about my food choices. Then, when I go to the party, I get a glass of wine, talk and don't have to worry about juggling a plate of food and a drink while having a conversation.

When I go to a gala, a banquet, a wedding or other planned event, I call ahead to speak to the person organizing the event, so I can speak directly with the chef. This is always the best help. You can tell pretty readily if a chef knows what he or she is talking about. Most chefs are aware of food allergies and restrictions these days and they will do anything they can to accommodate them. The problem with aware chefs is that many of them don't know how to cook flavorful foods without using butter, cream, sugar, cheese or flour. Even if you do not have a confirmed food allergy, if you know that gluten makes you depressed, tired, bloated, in pain or causes any other problem, you have the right to ask for no gluten in anything that you're consuming. There is no need to consume anything that makes you sick in this day and age. Most people in food services are acutely aware of this problem.

When someone invites me over to dinner, I talk to the host about my food restrictions before I go. Once, a friend of mine invited me to dinner. We had a long conversation about what I could and could not have. It was pretty simple, grilled or pan seared meat with vegetables. Make a salad with grilled fish or chicken, a honey mustard or balsamic dressing and lots of yummy vegetables. Perfect. Easy. Delicious.

When it came to the day of, the host called me and said she was panicking as to what to do and she decided to just do pizza. The kiss of death for someone like me who is allergic to both gluten and dairy. She actually said I should just bring my own dinner. I felt a combination of guilt for being a burden to her in her home and disregard for not being heard during our hour-long conversation in which she clearly seemed to get it. I Also felt disrespected for being told at the last minute that I would have to supply my own dinner when she was doing the inviting. I don't mind contributing to the party if that makes the host more comfortable, just tell me that sooner so I can get things together to share with others. I also don't mind eating before I go. The key is that I need to plan.

That evening I went to Whole Foods Market on the way and grabbed a couple of pieces of Grilled Salmon, steamed vegetables and a bottle of Balsamic salad dressing. I shared my fish and veggies with the other guests and discovered that the salad she made with chicken would have been plenty for me all along. It helps to ask specific questions of your host, especially if they are afraid of making you sick with their cooking. It is a valid concern of theirs and anything you can do to help them out is usually appreciated. Working with your host is a big help to both parties.

Eating this way can be very confusing to anyone that does it at the outset. You will have a period of adjustment as you take on this new way of life and others around you will have their own adjustment period trying to understand why you're no longer eating the way that they are. It can be astounding how personally other people take your changes. It is important to have support as you change and if you can get a friend or significant other to do this with you, this is the very best route. Accountability is super helpful.

Step Five: Eating while traveling or living in remote areas.

Traveling to other countries has its challenges when it comes to eating real organic food, especially if the country you're in has adopted many western ways of eating. Many countries in Asia and South America don't have strict laws on pesticide use, pollution, and food additives. Luckily, in many countries, they have plenty of fresh fruits and vegetables with many ways to prepare them. This is why people in third world countries are often healthier than we are in spite of their slack pollution standards and chemical exposures. They eat real food that they grow and prepare for themselves.

I worked with an American man living in Cambodia once. We did all our work over the internet using e-mail and Skype. He sent me pictures of menus from local restaurants that he frequented. I told him what to order and re-made a cleanse menu at a natural foods place into one that was specific to his needs. He had blood sugar and inflammatory bowel issues. I also looked up and read dozens of recipes from local traditions and modified them to remove the staple ingredient of sugar so that his cook, who comes once a week, could make these recipes for him at home.

Following these dietary suggestions would help him lose belly fat and his sugars would return to normal ranges. He couldn't figure out what was keeping him unhealthy as he was accustomed to eating fried foods, bread, and dairy products. When he cut those items out and focused on the suggestions that I recommended, his health improved. In many areas of the world, this isn't the easiest diet to follow but where there is a will for improved health, there typically is a way that I am going to help my clients find.

In many years of speaking to audiences at Whole Foods Market and working with clients, I have heard this same story over and over again; "I eat gluten here in the US and I get sick. I go to Europe and I can eat pasta in Italy, bread in France and pretty much anything I want without any reaction. For many years, the answer to why this phenomenon occurs was mainly conjecture. Now, we know why. Our wheat supply here in the US has been destroyed to the point of creating illness for most people that consume it.

In the book, Wheat Belly, by cardiologist Dr. William Davis he shares the history of the farming of wheat in the US. I highly recommend that you read his book as it is the best resource I have found to explain the gluten crisis that the US faces with allergies, Celiac disease, and gluten sensitivities on the rise every single day. In a nut shell, wheat has been scientifically manipulated through hybridization of the plant. It has been dramatically changed from the wheat that our grandparents consumed. The plant is nothing near what it used to be. In fact, they have manipulated wheat so much that it went from 14 chromosomes per plant to 28, doubling the gluten content, and making it suspect when it comes to why gluten is such an issue in the US.

If the genetically manipulated plants weren't enough, they also use a frightening technique to get the crops to ripen faster for harvest. You see, the grains don't all become ripe at the same time, so they saturate the crops with the herbicide Roundup (glyphosate, a known carcinogen and hormone disrupter) because they found that this poison makes the grains dry out for harvest. They then bleach the wheat grains with chlorine (another carcinogen), and use potassium bromate (yet another carcinogen) to help bread dough rise and hold together.

You may be wondering if all flour is treated this way and the answer is no, thankfully. If it says it's certified organic, it is not treated with these poisons. Often, ingredient labels will read; "unbleached and unbrominated flour." What that means is that those two processes aren't used but that does not mean that it is organic. Your best bet is to eat organic but, after a lot of research, I say don't eat gluten in the US *at all* unless it is Einkorn wheat or spelt. If you have an autoimmune disease or cancer, then no wheat should be consumed. I never thought I would be the person to say that, but the current research is overwhelmingly pointing to wheat as unsafe to consume.

The processing and farming of gluten uses multiple poisons. Eventually those grains become the flour used in most baked goods in the US. The ones to particularly pay attention to are the cheap goods with mile long ingredient lists. These products are found in convenience stores and mainstream grocery stores by the truckload. These foods increase your risk of cancer, diabetes and numerous other diseases. Please step away from the cheap, mass produced, heavily processed, wildly preserved, plastic wrapped and boxed baked goods. There are alternatives. Look for organic, preservative free, additive free, high quality baked goods. They will have a higher price tag but the long-term benefits to your health will be priceless (assuming your body can process wheat and other grains). The higher price tag is due to the quality of the product. It will help you appreciate them more and eat far less.

You're likely safe to consume wheat abroad in Europe because they do not allow the processing, the poisons nor the hybridization that we allow here in the US. The European Union has very strict standards for their food supply as do many other countries in the world that put the health of the people above the profits of the corporations.

A New Way of Eating

Most people I work with are perplexed as to how to change their diets. I get it. I was there once too. When my nutritionist told me in 1996 that I had to eliminate everything I was eating and start all over again to save my health, I was terrified. She handed me a few recipes and sent me to Whole Foods Market to get the ingredients. I walked into a Whole Foods for the first time and saw all the tiny boxes of things I absolutely did not recognize. I became overwhelmed, burst into tears and left the store. I then proceeded to lose 25 pounds in a very unhealthy way – starvation from not knowing what to eat.

I remember walking through the grocery store back then and feeling sad and disconnected from the foods I once loved. I also knew that if I ate any of them, the consequences were so great that I was dammed if I did. I was in a catch 22 and there were only one or two cookbooks with terrible recipes out on the shelves. I had to figure it out fast because there were no good resources and I had to eat.

It took me a while to understand this but eating a gluten free and dairy free diet is not about what breads, cakes, or cookies I could eat. Converting a poor diet made up mainly of wheat-based foods to gluten free options is not a solution for overall health. It was after I began to understand that the biggest gluten free and dairy free section in the grocery store is the produce area that my health truly turned around for the best.

Eventually I would teach cooking classes at the largest Whole Foods Market in Los Angeles. Classes were held in the produce department. I would have everyone turn around and look at all the fruits and vegetables and I would say; "Look at this section. Everything you see here is gluten free and dairy free. There are endless combinations of recipes you can create in this section alone. When you focus your diet in this department, your health will dramatically improve, and in most cases, your chronic conditions will heal."

What to Do
Now that you know one of the biggest secrets to getting well

(eating real food), what do you do next? How do you find the time to make this happen?

First off, create a plan for your health through food. This is where mindset comes in. Without making up your mind that you will do this, you probably won't. To help you make that decision, think about how you will feel, what you will look like, how much energy you will have and how much younger you will appear once you adopt this new way of eating. Picture yourself being able to get out of bed with a healthy body to carry you through your day. Imagine what it will feel like to have your symptoms disappear one by one. Envision yourself as you desire to be, make the changes necessary to achieve that and set about making that happen. This is an "all in" participation goal. You can do it!

You may be thinking that you are a terrible cook, or you don't like to cook or that you don't have time. All those things may be true, but do they have to be? There was a time that I was considered the worst cook in my family but then I ended up becoming a celebrity chef and writing a cookbook and an online program with recipes I developed for my celebrity chef clients. I grew up cooking at a very early age, but I still wasn't great at it until I had to save my health. In order to do that, I had to figure it out and make it work. There were so many kitchen failures and timing disasters but over time, I became world class at cooking. You can too.

Everything you learn to do well must start with doing it. Practicing it over and over again is how you get good at anything. Eating is an absolute necessity. If you want to stay healthy for a long time, cooking your own food made from whole ingredients from the Earth is the very best way. Learning to cook your own food is such an incredible way to connect with your own health and wellness. It is such a sensual experience, taking in the colors visually, chopping the fruits and vegetables, breathing in the aromas as they cook together then sharing the meal with loved ones as you savor all the delicious flavors.

You will get in a rhythm that works for you. You can have music playing while you cook or a TV show or podcast on that you like. You can have your significant other, roommate, or kids help you, so everything goes more quickly. If you have left overs, that you are afraid might spoil, you can put them in containers in the freezer to have for the next week or for a night when you just don't feel like cooking.

The Bottom Line on Eating This Way

Eating a diet like what I have outlined in this chapter can reverse or eliminate many of the chronic conditions that people are suffering from. I have personally seen the following diseases and symptoms reversed, healed, or arrested with the type of diet I have been making for clients, friends, family and myself for over two decades now.

Alzheimer's
Diabetes
Irritable Bowel Syndrome
Fibromyalgia
Chronic Fatigue Syndrome
Hashimoto's Thyroiditis
Ulcers
Cancer
Benign Tumors
Liver Disease
Arthritis
Depression
Bi-Polar Disorder
Chronic Sinusitis
Diverticulitis
Colitis
Multiple Sclerosis
Heart Disease

Autism

Kidney Disease

Food is the holy grail of wellness in most cases. Some diseases need much more than food for true and lasting healing. They need exercise, proper sleep, supplementation, herbal medicine and the power of the mind to help you heal. The mind section of this book will go more in depth to assist you in understanding that food simply supports your body to heal itself. The mind and spirit do the actual healing. More about that in the second half of the book.

Illness is a wakeup call. You have free will which means you have choices. You can answer the call and take your healing into your own hands, you can ignore what is happening to your body, or you can knowingly push aside the pain until it comes to critical mass and you must do something to get well. When this happens, it is often too late. It's much harder to reverse the list of diseases I just mentioned once they have reached the acute stage. In many cases you may never be able to. The sooner you take care of the problem, the sooner you can heal and get well. It is much easier to stay well than to get well. It will take every ounce of your energy to do so. It is ALL up to you. My professional and personal recommendation is not to wait.

Please decide now that you are willing to Get Well Now. It is the first and most important step you will take. You are not alone in this journey. You don't have to be. I am here. My community called Get Well Now is here. Please join us in our private Facebook community. All you have to do is ask to be a part of it. It is a place for positive support, to ask questions, share stories and provide solutions for healing you in mind, body and soul.

You've got this! You can get well. You've got help. Just take one step towards it now. It will be the best thing you ever did for you. I promise!

Maintaining This Lifestyle

So many people have an enormously difficult time maintaining a lifestyle of real food, chemical free. There are many reasons for this. One big one is that these foods are not readily available in most parts of the US. There is a marked difference between the east and west coasts of the US in terms of available, clean, organic food. In California, there are farmer's markets all year round, grocery stores have a much larger selection of organic produce, and restaurant menus have multiple choices for fresh menu items without cheese, cream or wheat. It is so much easier to live an organic, fresh life there.

On the east coast, even in a major city like DC, where I am from, there are very small organic produce sections in grocery stores. Even Trader Joe's and Whole Foods Market have far fewer choices than California. Menu items in restaurants routinely have cheese, heavy dressings and sugary items like dates, cranberries, pears, and honey pecans (often dusted with wheat flour by the way) that are inflammation producing – and by inflammation, I also mean weight and illness producing. These things go hand in hand.

I find that in more affluent areas, like the Hamptons, you have access to restaurants that are farm to table, organic produce, juice bars and organic, conscious living. It is a sign of the more educated and wealthy population having access to better, more healthy foods. It is definitely a situation of demographics, but I don't consistently find that people with high incomes have a better grasp on food that is truly healthy. They just have the means to afford the best possible.

The second biggest road block to living an organic, clean food kind of lifestyle is expense. This is where I get into discussions with people on a regular and continuing basis. Corporate conglomerate food companies have done an incredibly effective job of marketing to the masses and literally brainwashing them into believing that their foods are safe when there is overwhelming evidence that shows that it simply is not true. The real truth is that even if the conventional broccoli costs $2.39 and the organic broccoli sitting right next to it is $2.69, most people won't pay the thirty-cent difference. They do not see the value and they do not know that eating conventional produce will cost you far, far, more in the long run. The purse strings now are more pressing than the disease yet to come because there is a massive disconnect between the two. It is in this gap that these food corporations get you to say yes to cheap foods now without caring one little bit that you will pay dearly later.

I laid this all out for you in a previous chapter, but I want to reiterate this, when you swallow poison every single day in "food" that lacks the nutrition the body needs, you set yourself up for a chronic illness that will cost you far more over the long haul in the loss of your health, the loss of your job, and the loss of your life. Those things cannot be replaced. And the sad truth is that most people won't do anything about their diets until the extreme diagnosis comes. I know this one first hand because I was naïve enough to think that after I healed irritable bowel syndrome, ulcers, migraines, and frequent debilitating muscle spasms in my late twenties that I could return to my old ways of eating gluten, dairy, sugar, soy, food chemicals, and pesticide laden produce on occasion and still be just fine and the truth was, I was completely wrong. I got much sicker when I did, and I ended up testing positive for Mixed Connective Tissue Disease, Fibromyalgia, and Chronic Fatigue Syndrome. The diseases just became more catastrophic and the management of their symptoms became far more difficult.

I tell you this, not to scare you but to let you know that once you are sick, you cannot consume a food substance that you know does you harm. Your very best bet is to change your habits permanently and to commit to being dedicated to your health and wellbeing by eating foods that you know nourish your body to heal itself because that is what the body is designed to do. Once you really get this, you will be home free. In most cases, you will be healthy, whole and well.

When you read the mind section, you will get a lot more in maintaining this way of eating. So much of it is mindset. It has to do with personal development and evolution. This is the key to losing weight and keeping it off. It is with your mind that you truly grow and change. If you don't change your inner world, your outer world won't change in a lasting way, and you won't be able to maintain these dietary changes.

There are ten tips that can help you in terms of forming good habits and maintaining this way of eating.

Tip #1 – Plan your meals each week.

Tip #2 – Eat before you go to an event.

Tip #3 – Focus on what you can have, not what you can't.

Tip #4 – Learn to cook and prepare your own meals.

Tip #5 – Shop the outer ring of the grocery store.

Tip #6 – Pay close attention to food quality & choose the best.

Tip #7 – Don't let yourself get overly hungry.

Tip #8 – Keep nuts and/or seeds on hand everywhere you go.

Tip #9 – Before you eat something you know will make you sick, go over the consequences in your head.

Tip #10 – Set on the path of self-love and everything becomes easier for you.

The Best Science

I tell my clients and community that your body is your own laboratory. It is constantly giving you feedback about what works for you and what does not. Our body chemistries are all different. What works for you may not work for the person sitting next to you. We each have our own way of processing food, emotions, thoughts, beliefs, and the energy in and around us. We are all unique.

Because we are all different, there isn't a scientific experiment that could come close to the needs of your specific body chemistry. You are your own laboratory. So, start to think of yourself this way. Subtract a food ingredient like gluten for a couple of weeks and watch how your body reacts when you add it back it. Your body is giving you feedback all the time. Begin to listen to what it is telling you.

I always tell my clients not to wait for a scientific experiment to tell you what works or does not. Science is always at least twenty years ahead of western medicine adopting something on a large scale. Meanwhile, you don't have to become a statistic because you chose not to figure things out on your own, in your personal laboratory.

There is so much information available to us today. There are incredible doctors and wellness professionals that are studying the leading-edge science (including me) that are interested in your health more than chasing dollars from big food and pharma. Find a leader in the field who resonates with you – or many of them – and learn from their wisdom and experience.

Ultimately, you will learn in this book about listening not only to your body but to your own internal sense of knowing what is best for you. You are not stuck. You are free to conduct your own experiments to find out what works for you. Food is the very best place to start. Adopt a lifestyle of food choices that work for you. You will know how well your lifestyle is working for you by how great you look and feel.

Cheers to your great health and creating your own delicious, healthy, and satisfying new way of eating. You will be so happy with your new choices. They will make everything better for you and your family!

PART II

THE POWER OF THE MIND

The mind is more powerful than most people can fathom. The most extraordinary things have been accomplished through simply one thing, changing your mind. Focus, dedication and setting your mind to achieve a specific result carries more power than anything else on the planet because within it, you are wielding the greatest asset you have – the ability to choose a different thought and to create an entirely different outcome than the one in front of you.

Everything that was ever created started with a thought. This book was, at one time, just a thought in my head of something I wanted to create and share. The building you are sitting in right now was originally a thought. Action was taken in order to put the pieces of the structure together, starting with the foundation. It took many people to make that building a reality but, again, it all started with a thought.

A series of decisions made on your own behalf is what will get you well. You must take action to follow your decisions while fueling them with your passion, determination, and will if you want to be better than you were before. We live in a pill swallowing world that constantly tells us that our healing is not in our hands. It is given over to doctors to decide what is best for us and while they are trained professionals, there's one thing they don't have and that's the experience of what it is like to be you in mind, body and soul. They don't know what you think about, the choices you make, and the way your body feels on a regular basis. Western medical doctors are trained to diagnose your problem and treat it with pharmaceutical drugs, surgery, and in some very specific instances, food (diabetes, heart disease, high cholesterol to name a few). They are amazing people, doing necessary work but they only cover one piece of the pie of health while keeping you in the sickness model of care through specifically treating symptoms, not underlying causes.

The deeper problem is that most people don't really know themselves. Some of you reading this book may have a very deep understanding of self and a profound connection to your body, mind and soul. For you, this section is a reminder because we can all use that. For many of us though, we have little idea of the mind/body/soul connection and could use some advice on strengthening the connections between them but first, we need to learn how to recognize and work with them.

This section of the book will cover how to connect the body with the mind and the even more critical part of it all. It's the part that does the actual healing and while it sounds nebulous, stick with me here. I will help make this a concrete for you with exercises you can do to make a connection between the holistic parts of yourself – mind, body, and soul/energy field.

7

WHAT YOU MUST DO FIRST

Years ago, when MySpace was a thing, I received a question from a Ph.D. physicist completing his doctoral dissertation at USC in computer science. He wanted to know, "What is the soul?" It is a profound question that I had, at that point spent nearly a decade and my Ph.D. in Transpersonal Psychology pondering. I never forgot the discussion we had and now I have a lifelong friend and great conversation to share that started with a scientist examining the nature of the soul with me.

The answer went something like this; The soul is the energy that animates you. It is the only thing that you cannot live without. It carries within it your mission and purpose in life. It knows what you came here to complete and work through. Your soul contains your skills, talents, abilities, interests, and gifts that you bring to share with the world.

The soul runs on love, compassion, kindness, joy, excitement, caring, and all things that are light, bright, and beautiful. Imagine for a moment, that your soul brings you experiences that are meant to show you what you aren't, so you can become who you are meant to be. I think of your soul as your teacher, your personality is your student and you are in Earth school (a term coined by Gary Zukav in his book, Seat of the Soul), learning the lessons that life has to show you in only the way that you are meant to learn them. Since you have free will, granted to your personality, you can remain fully unconscious to the power and intention of your soul for your entire lifetime or you can choose to become a partner with your soul to reach the highest potential you can for your life. It is ALL up to YOU.

You are the student taking classes in The School of Life and you keep repeating the same classes over and over again, especially in your relationships. Those are some of the hardest classes The School of Life has to offer. The one class that will ask you to become aware of your soul, more than any other class you will have, is "Wake-up Call 101". The wake-up call will come to you in many different ways throughout your lifetime. The first time it comes as an adult, in a loud and clear way is often between the ages of 27-30. It may come at any time and most of us have multiple wake-up calls.

One way you may be asked to wake up to the power of your soul is through illness. A diagnosis of a chronic illness, deemed by western medicine as something you will have for your entire life while having you take medication with massive potential side effects including death, is where most people will sit in this class. They will feel doomed to stay in this class for the rest of their lives (which may be dramatically shortened by their dis-ease and medications), because *a doctor told them this is true for them.*

So, how do you graduate from this class? How can you pass a class that is so potentially bleak? What if you have cancer? Diabetes? Autoimmune diseases like arthritis, MS, or ALS? What then?!?!? Here is the BIG SECRET. Here is the way to pass the class and get to the next level. Choose it.

This is what you must do first. You have a power that is beyond measure. You have the ability to CHOOSE your way up and out of so many situations you never, ever, thought you could. The first thing you do is decide. This decision must be definitive.

You must decide with every single, cell, atom, and molecule of your body that you are going to get well. You're not going to buy into what the doctors are telling you and you are going to make different choices for your own wellbeing. You are going to make the most powerful move of your life. *You are going to take YOUR healing into YOUR own hands.* This is THE way out of this misery you are in and YOU are the only person that can create this experience.

When you are ready to choose, and you've made that decision, the next step is to find someone who has had and healed (or completely arrested the development of their disease). When you find this person or group of people, talk to them. Get to know the steps they took and follow them. Know that you are going to need to hire help to get you through this and it probably won't be covered by insurance. Part of getting truly well is to step outside of exclusively using the western medical model and carve out a path that is right for you. To do this, you will follow your gut instinct, allowing your love for you to lead you, as opposed to following the fear to do what everyone else does, while remaining ill and on drugs that potentially cause horrific side effects.

It will be super important to give up the idea that someone else should pay for your wellness. It will take a team of healers to get you well and it will cost you far less than you could possibly imagine in the long run. Western medcine is focused on suppressing symptoms and often, does not look for the root cause of your illness.

I was only 27 when I discovered the path to wellness. It is when my wake-up call came to me in the form of multiple illnesses and unexplained experiences. I was so tormented by all the pain I was in on all levels of my being – physical, mental, emotional, and spiritual. It was a truly horrific time in my personal history. Now, at 50 years old, I can look back to see that it was the most powerful thing I ever, ever, ever, did and I would not change a thing about the path I took to get well, not even the cost, which was upwards of $75,000.00 over a period of two decades. That comes to $312.00 a month over a twenty-year period, which for a woman who is single and lived on an erratic income in one of the most expensive cities in the world while still managing to write six books, co-author two more, become a celebrity chef, have a private transpersonal therapy practice, network like crazy, host a radio show and podcast series, and speak around the country, that is pretty darned good. And please understand that my education is factored into that number.

The point is you can do this work very inexpensively and very effectively out of pocket. The tradeoff of excellent health will be worth every minute and every penny. I know this one first hand. I know without question that if I had not taken my healing into my own hands that fateful moment in 1996, I would have died of cancer. I was quickly headed for that kind of catastrophic diagnosis with all the risk factors I had and with eating all the wrong foods that tore up my intestinal tract – which must be healed in order to be healthy.

To give you an idea of the risk factors I was up against; When my mom was pregnant with me, she was prescribed a drug that was given to women routinely to prevent miscarriages between 1938 and 1971. Mom had already miscarried another child less than a year before she became pregnant with me though many women were given the drug even if they weren't at risk of miscarrying. The drug was diethylstilbestrol, also known as the DES hormone. It was the first synthetic estrogen drug ever created and prescribed on a mass level. In the generations of daughters born to mothers that took the drug, there is a high rate of certain kinds of uterine and breast cancers as well as infertility and, you guessed it, miscarriages. I personally suffered one miscarriage when I was married then never got pregnant again.

DES has come to be known as the silent thalidomide. In case you're not aware of what that drug did to babies in utero, it caused a wide variety of birth defects, mainly limb deformities. It was used to alleviate morning sickness. DES was and is still not as well-known as thalidomide though millions of women were given the drug. The side effects are not noticeable like a child with no hands would be. We silently suffer with cancers and never being able to fulfill the dream of being mothers and that is what happened to me, one failed pregnancy and no others to follow.

The second cancer risk factor I had was at birth when my mom was told not to breast feed me. It was a popular belief in the 1960's that breast feeding was not necessary. My mom had breast fed my eldest sister for a short time, but she developed an infection of the mammary ducts called mastitis. At the time doctors told these patients to stop breast feeding immediately and don't breast feed any future children. I was the third child.

The link between babies that weren't breast fed and chronic illness down the road is undeniable. There are certain immunities that babies get from the breast milk that help to populate the intestinal tract with healthy bacteria that will assist the immune system in fighting off illness throughout our lives. Without this first line of defense, we become susceptible to infections throughout childhood and beyond that can eventually evolve into chronic illnesses.

The next risk factor I have for cancers were scoliosis screenings I had every four months for four years during high school. I had one of the top orthopedic surgeons in the nation at National Orthopedic Hospital. My doctor was the orthopedist for the Washington Redskins. In the DC area, it could not get any better than that. Women that had these screenings have been put at a high risk for breast cancer due to the radiation exposure.

The next risk factor is the one that most doctors don't tell you about because they simply either don't know, don't have time to learn about, or won't look at the connection between the mind and the body. This is the risk factor of trauma sustained during childhood and betrayal experiences (and that is what childhood trauma typically is). The Adverse Childhood Experiences Study (ACE Study) is the largest public health study ever done that most people – not even doctors – know about. The ones that do often refute the findings.

The ACE Study has followed over seventeen thousand patients at Kaiser Permanente in San Diego, California from 1995 to present. They asked patients a series of questions about their childhood, creating the ACE Quiz. It's a simple ten question quiz that covers different types of abuse – physical, sexual, and emotional. It also covers different types of family dysfunction – divorce, death or abandonment of a parent, mental illness in a parent, alcoholism/drug addiction of a parent, incarceration of a parent, watching one parent beat the other. When you take the quiz, you tally your score. Those with scores of four or more are more likely to develop chronic illnesses that dramatically shorten their lifespans than those that did not have so much dysfunction and abuse.

One of the top diseases seen in those with high ACE scores is cancer. My score indicated that my risk for chronic diseases were much higher than normal. I was physically, sexually, and emotionally abused as a child which also added to my cancer risk.

It has been found that cancer diagnoses typically happen after a crisis like a cheating spouse, the death of someone close, the betrayal of a dear friend, or some other instance where there is a huge emotional upheaval that is often coupled with the buildup of long term resentment.

I had the opportunity to give a talk to a room full of oncologists. An oncologist friend of mine invited me to speak at a gathering in which he was speaking about being more conservative in offering chemo therapy to patients. He asked me to talk about my story of being struck by lightning as well as the emotional connection that I have seen in my clients over the years associated with illness. I was shocked that of the doctors in the room, none of them, had any idea that their patients likely had a precipitating emotional event prior to diagnosis.

I shared with them this wasn't something I just noticed. It was a very strong link that is documented repeatedly. I was shocked and saddened that these doctors, many of whom were considered the best in the business were unaware of this fundamental link. Some of the doctors were fascinated while others were stone faced, arms crossed in front of their hearts, not welcoming in the possibility that cancer was anything other than a physical disease.

I tell you this to begin to illustrate to you what is perhaps the largest contributing factor to disease, the mental and emotional fallout from trauma and betrayal experiences in which you feel that the life has been drained from you by way of someone close to you or some traumatic event that changed your life. The mind is an incredibly powerful instrument of both healing and potential destruction. It is quite possibly the most important asset you have.

My most recent cancer risk was being struck by lightning. There is a higher risk for melanoma and carcinomas in people who were struck by lightning. I have been advised to watch moles closely for discoloration and migration.

8

MORE THAN JUST MINDSET

Everywhere you look, personal development experts are talking about mindset. They discuss how to train your mind to erase subconscious programming, think differently, focus on what you want to achieve, and create the life you desire with your thoughts. I don't know about you but reading that last sentence is exhausting because it takes a lot of brain power to think your way out of or into anything, especially illness.

I often say that when you change our mind, you also change your life. But changing your mind isn't always that easy. There tends to be a road an individual takes to get to the point of decision. That road can take many years of reversing the thinking that got you into the situation you're in.

One of my earliest mentors in healing, over two decades ago is Dr. Caroline Myss. I think she really nailed it in her work in the eighties and nineties when she said that healing has to do with getting as much of your thinking (your energy) into the present moment as possible. In order to do that, she says we have to "call our spirits back" from past experiences in which they left us as happens when trauma occurs.

All shamanic traditions have the ceremony of bringing "soul

pieces" back into the body for the body, mind and soul to heal. Even thousands of years ago, it was understood that illness was not just physical. It encompassed the whole being. Systems were created in ancient times that focused on the energy system of the human body as paramount to healing the physical body. Two such recognizable systems are the chakra system from the ancient Vedic traditions of India and the Chinese system of the meridians, or energy pathways, that are associated with the major organ systems of the body, used in Chinese medicine. These systems are now known as The Human Energy System.

Today, these systems are still being used worldwide to assist practitioners in diagnosing and treating illnesses of all kinds through acupuncture and Ayurvedic medicine. Many practitioners in holistic medicine use a combination of these ancient medical methodologies to assist in diagnosis and treatment of illnesses. Now, there are many western medical doctors' training in functional medicine, acupuncture, osteopathy, and various other holistic medical approaches as they return to what practitioners have known for thousands of years; when the different parts of holistic system are engaged, healing happens naturally and rapidly. Maintaining these parts of the self leads to lasting, sustained health.

Back when I studied these ideas, they always resonated with me. Perhaps it was because of all the traumas I experienced from an early age, but I felt in my core there was something to the concept of bringing your energy back into your body from past experiences. I think this was due to always having a feeling that I didn't have the ability to focus on things in my every day experience. I always felt disconnected and not a part of the world around me. I was constantly in fight or flight mode, waiting for the next dramatic moment to unfold in my daily life.

In the two decades since learning about The Human Energy System, I have come to believe that having our spirits stuck in past experiences of trauma is absolutely the case, with precision and certainty. Not only have I experienced this to be truth within my own life, I have also helped hundreds of others experience the exact same phenomena. And honestly, it really comes down to one thing; forgiveness. Another great word I like to use instead of forgiveness comes from one of the incomparable founders of Mind/Body Medicine, Dr. Joan Borysenko; Release-ness. Isn't that a great way to think about it? You are releasing your emotional burdens and in the action of forgiving you become lighter and freer, with more energy to run your everyday experience.

Your ability to release the power that you have allowed past experiences of betraying self and others, is where the key to healing lies. It is inside of you and only you can let go of what is keeping you in the mind loop of detrimental patterns that are likely contributing to your illness.

This all sounds good but it's easier said than done. I have found that having a guide help you through this kind of deep seated emotional patterning and the attached beliefs that are draining you of your precious energy is really necessary. I am not talking about talk therapy. I am talking about finding the method of releasing deep emotional belief patterns from your biology so that you can come into the present moment in a way that you never have before; especially if you have suffered trauma and betrayal.

There are a number of different therapies that are available to help you with releasing stuck emotions and patterns. Here are a few:

- Ro-Hun Therapy
- Inner Child Therapy
- Energy Work (Reiki, The Radiance Technique, Healing Touch)
- Cranial Sacral Therapy
- Shamanic Soul Retrieval Work

- Eye Movement Desensitization and Reprocessing (EMDR)
- Emotional Freedom Technique (EFT)
- Spiritual Psychotherapy
- Whole Person Integration Technique

There are many more methods out there than the ones I have listed. These are ones that I am very familiar with and have tried on myself or have used on my clients with incredible, lasting results.

Here are some clues that you may not be in the present and may need to bring your energy back through some sort of transpersonal therapy:

- You feel spacy, unfocused and distracted easily.
- You feel disconnected like you're not "in your body"
- You may feel disconnected from one side of your body or the other (almost as if you don't feel it).
- You startle easily and it's hard to recover from it.
- You ruminate over past events, focusing on anger, sadness, jealousy, or unworthiness on a regular, often daily basis.
- You become obsessively fearful.
- You have nightmares and/or night terrors or talk in your sleep or sleep walk on a regular basis.
- You think about a trauma you went through on a regular basis, playing the story over in your head.
- You cut people off whom you love without notice or discussion.
- You are paranoid that others are talking about you or are out to get you in some way.
- You have extreme anxiety.
- You can't remember very much, if anything about your childhood or all you do remember are bad memories.

- You may be very quick to anger or sadness that is out of proportion to the situation.
- You blow up at others and/or throw tantrums.
- You drink alcohol, do drugs, eat, shop, have sex/porn excessively, watch TV, or you're online excessively to avoid your feelings.
- You either can't identify what you're feeling or your over identify with your feelings – sometimes vacillating between the two.
- You have extreme anxiety every day over just about everything or one thing in particular.

If you identify with many of these symptoms, you may want to pursue some kind of spiritual psychotherapy work. Search around, talk to others like your setting out on a trip in a foreign land where you get to explore the things that interest you. Be curious, get referrals, read books, google methods you hear about, interview therapists, and above all, trust that you will find precisely what is right for you. Don't think it will be a bed of roses, which if you think about it, can be dangerous and thorn filled. Think of all the wonderful and all the awful on your path to getting well are the pieces and parts you're meant to experience in your efforts to heal.

With everyone that I have known along the way that truly healed and sustained that healing, there was always a spiritual component. I'm not just talking about the people I have worked with. I am also referring the amazing healers I met along the way; best-selling authors and major health and wellness influencers. People that overcame their own illnesses to help millions ALWAYS, always, had a spiritual component to their wellness pathways. Some were religious, some were spiritual, some were nature oriented, some were highly logical people who came to understand there is some power that is unseen that helps the body to heal. It is this power that will get you well. It is more than just a matter of you changing your mind, it is a matter of your spiritual growth. It isn't separate from your body. It is all one and when you focus on calling your precious energy back from the heartaches and betrayals you've experienced, you release resentment. That releases your biology from the enslavement of illness. You have the power to do this. The question is how.

9

ACTIVELY CHANGING YOUR MIND

You've been introduced to the idea of bringing your energy back into your body to bring healing to your cells. Perhaps you've heard about this concept before, but it sounded too out there for you to grasp. Maybe it's resonating with you now that it has been explained in some sort of logical way. I just ask that you give it a chance to see if perhaps this is the thing you've been looking for. Healing is not just physical, it is beyond the physical.

A simple way to relate to the concept of energy returning to your body to heal its cells is the feeling you get in a moment of realization. This common experience, best known as the "aha moment" has an associated physical feeling of a shift that can best be described as something has lifted from you and now there's room in your worldview for a different understanding than you had the moment just prior to your realization.

The kind of work I recommend for wellness is essentially invoking multiple "aha moments" repeatedly. Think for a moment about what that must feel like. That sense of getting lighter, freer, and more aware rapidly is the best way to describe what calling your energy back from the experiences that are draining you; often without your awareness or consent as SO MUCH of it is unconscious.

Psychospiritual work brings what is unconscious and damaging you to the conscious part of your mind while simultaneously releasing energy you may never need be consciously aware of. The result is that you cannot explain why you are no longer attached to a specific reaction. You just are, and you are free because of it.

Releasing the Pain

Our emotions will run us if we allow them to. For most of us, we will lay victim to them for our entire lives. With the hundreds of clients, I have worked with, I have found that each person has a particular set of dark, self-defeating thoughts and their associated feelings. There is a pathway each person takes as they cycle through well-worn patterns over and over again. At the core tends to be one emotion that they always arrive upon and that is their addictive emotion. For some it's anger, for others it's sadness, for others it's shame, hopelessness, unworthiness, and so on.

Most people think of those emotions as 'negative emotions'. That label automatically shames the emotion, making it wrong for its very existence. The natural tendency would be to push it way, turn your back on it, and bury it with any number of distractions that keep you from feeling the negative emotion you want nothing more than to avoid.

After working with emotions for so long, I have come to see them not as 'negative emotions' but as teaching emotions. I believe these emotions hold the keys to clearing every pattern, and ultimately to your health and wellness. These emotions have come to you to teach you something about who you really are. They want the same thing that you do; they want to be seen, heard, understood, and loved.

How do you love these broken and beaten down parts of you?

Well first, you must learn to listen to them. That means you must stop running from them. There are myriad ways we run from our emotions. The most typical ways are with numbing mechanisms like the following:

- Alcohol/drugs/cigarettes
- Sugar or starchy foods (food addiction)
- Excessive attachment to romance
- Sex/porn
- Co-dependent relationships (love addiction)
- Excessive TV
- Excessively online/phone
- Excessive shopping
- Constantly talking
- Excessive exercise
- Workaholism
- Excessive lying
- Excessive video game playing

As you look at this list, see which things you may be doing to excess, even if it's only on weekends or other binge worthy times. Think about the things that people say to you most about what they see as an excessive activity of yours. Does your husband complain that you talk too much, and others agree? Does your wife say you're at work too much? These criticisms can be clues that you are using something to excess to avoid feelings you don't want to feel.

Begin to notice the ways you numb yourself. You will see a definite pattern as you focus on this. You may find that you run out the door to go shopping when someone or something upsets you. You may get angry at someone and think, "I need a drink or a cigarette!". You may run to the kitchen and indulge in something you know will make you feel sick or emotionally worse.

Notice the emotion that is triggered and which one you cycle through on a regular basis. See the pattern first before you begin to work with it. Let yourself go to the thing you use to numb yourself with and allow it to happen. Observe yourself as though you are in a laboratory. What are you thinking and feeling during the whole cycle? What kinds of things do you do to repress your feelings? Do you become over emotional or emotionally cut off? All these things are clues to help you work through your emotions and will be fodder for you in processing them.

Once you determine the emotions you cycle through on a regular basis, narrow them down to the one emotion you use most regularly. You will have one. Perhaps it's sadness and you cry at any and everything. Perhaps it's anger and everything pisses you off. What you're looking for is where you end up on a regular basis when things go south in your life.

Greeting Your Emotional Addiction

Once you have identified the emotion you cycle down to most of the time, write it down. Think about the situation at hand and write down all the emotions that come up for you. If you're having trouble identifying emotions in general, it can be helpful to reference the following list.

Anger
Rage
Hopelessness
Fearful
Abandoned
Sadness
Frustrated
Anxious
Unworthy
Horrified
Disgusted
Discouraged

Grief
Alarmed
Confused
Distrustful
Controlling
Judgmental
Jealous
Numb
Shameful
Victimized
Lost
Isolated
Lonely
Insecure
Discouraged
Disconnected
Desperate

You get the idea that there are a range of emotions you can be experiencing at any given moment. Sometimes, you feel a number of them simultaneously. In the case of both confusion and anxiety, I have found with numerous clients that these two emotions are a mixture of emotions colliding. You may want to spend some time sorting out which emotions are causing your confusion or anxiety.

Often when you experience an emotion, it will come out as a thought like, "I feel like I can't do anything right". This thought has emotions attached to it so ask yourself, "When I think this thought, how do I feel?" This question gets you closer to the emotion. Perhaps you feel unworthy when you think you can't do anything right. Perhaps you feel sadness or frustration or fear. Listen and feel so you can begin to be in touch with your emotions. Even if you're more in the category of over emotional, you may not be in touch with your emotional inner life. You may just be re-acting unconsciously all the time and have little idea why you feel the way you do but you know your life is a mess because of it. Or, perhaps you have an idea, but you just don't know how to overcome the pattern.

Until you begin to learn your patterns and to isolate the emotions attached to the thoughts, *you will be a slave to them.* They control you in an unconscious way and the people closest to you will suffer from your lack of emotional consciousness. This is especially true if you experienced a childhood with traumas and emotionally stunted parents who constantly modeled their own lack of emotional maturity and intelligence.

One of the greatest gifts you can give yourself is the awareness of your emotions. When you begin this process, you begin to emerge from the bottom of yourself, like the Phoenix rising from the ashes, you will become lighter, freer, happier, and more loving. This happens because you begin to truly and deeply love yourself through loving the most unlovable parts of you – your so called "negative" emotions.

Whole Person Integration Technique

As I mentioned previously in this chapter, begin to think of your negative emotions as teaching emotions. They are here to teach you about who you really are. They want the same thing you do, to be loved, cared for, heard, seen, understood, and forgiven for the things they are doing to hold you back from the best you.

The first book I was published in was an anthology of women entrepreneurs who were making a difference in the world. It was called, *Inspiration to Realization, Volume III.* I contributed a chapter to this book in the section on spiritual growth. In this chapter, I gave readers my Whole Person Integration Technique (WPIT) which is a holistic process that helps you identify, love, and release these broken parts of you. At the time, I called the process, Emotional Alchemy.

This technique gives you simple instructions on how to identify the emotion that is currently stopping you, learn the thoughts the emotion believes, learn where it is located in your body, and it gives you a simple process on how to release the emotion from your body.

I have been using this process and its inspiration from my Transpersonal Psychology program, Ro-Hun Therapy, to help people genuinely heal emotional addictions and patterns for nearing fifteen years now. What I have found repeatedly, when the client does the work it takes to identify and release these stuck emotions is that, after doing this process, their realities change. What used to emotionally trigger them, no longer does so.

Marlene's Story

When Marlene showed up to work with me, she was being run by a number of emotions. The one she cycled through regularly was sadness. She cried over nearly everything and was labeled by everyone as being "overly sensitive". She resented that label and felt victimized on a regular basis by everyone around her in some way.

As we dug deeper, we found that she had been sexually abused by multiple people as a child, criticized regularly by her parents and teachers, lost in the shuffle of a big family, raped as a teen ager, ridiculed by her siblings, and she routinely took responsibility for every wrong that was ever done to her.

Because of the way that she stuffed her emotions, she became very ill in her teens and twenties and received a cascade of disease diagnoses. She was essentially imploding because she had taken on the role of victim and she had adopted a self-perception that caused her to feel zero self-regard. Her lack of self-respect came directly from believing she was only worthy of being beaten up, used and discarded. She had no idea who she was or the power she had available to her to heal herself.

To assist her to get well, she needed to learn to drop the perception that she was always the victim. She needed to learn the ways that she had contributed to her own demise and how her teaching emotions were driving her ever towards illness and self-deprecation. She also needed to understand how she had victimized herself through turning her anger in on herself.

We first worked with her diet to help detoxify her body and to help support her while we did the emotional work. She was being unconsciously run by the following emotions:

1. Resentment
2. Fear
3. Anxiety
4. Sadness
5. Jealousy
6. Shame
7. Unworthiness

We worked with each emotion, where they were located in her body, what shape they took, what they believed, thought, and felt and how they were tied to the Human Energy System and its attributes. As she began to love and release these parts of the self, her body healed, her mind healed, and her spirit was able to soar.

When she had all that energy available to her, she became the things she had secretly wanted to be. She became successful in every endeavor she set out to achieve. In releasing the emotions, where they were in her body, their deep-seated negative beliefs, and gaining love and compassion for them, she got well. Now, when she feels any of the above seven emotions that used to weigh her down, she can process them herself or seek my help when things get tough.

This is an incredibly important thing to understand. Though the emotions hold the key to your healing and personal evolution, when you release them, it does not mean that you will never feel them again. What it means is that your relationship to them and how you once perceived them will change. Part of being human is dealing with difficult emotions and experiences. You won't be turned into some automaton who feels nothing – that would be ridiculous. You just become adept at working with them to get well.

The Human Energy System

I mentioned in the last section that you have an energy system and that each part of that system has attributes associated with them. Each part correlates to the physical body and to your emotional and mental states. There are seven major centers of this energy system based in thousands of years of study and use. Countless practitioners have found the value of using the energy system as a means for healing and I completely concur. I could not have been as effective as a practitioner if I did not have the deep study and use of this system.

A wonderful book that outlines the Human Energy System and its attributes that I recommend to every client I have had because of its intelligent, logical, and modern-day applications, is *Anatomy of The Spirit* by Caroline Myss. I mentioned Dr. Myss as one of my early mentors when I began my healing pathway over twenty years ago. I recommend reading her book for more depth and understanding of your energy system. For now, I will provide a brief outline so you can begin to see the parts and attributes that may help you put a few things together with your own health.

The Seven Centers of The Human Energy System

1ˢᵗ Center:
Located at the base of the spine, this center is associated with earthly life. It is your connection to the planet, to your family, to society at large. This center is your presence in the world, how you show up, but also, how you're generally perceived by others.

Energetic Drain: Struggle of all kinds/fear/worry over safety

Archetypes:
Unhealthiest Expression: The Wounded Soldier
Healthiest Expression: The Earth Mother

Diseases Associated with The 1ˢᵗ Center:
Hemorrhoids, vaginal problems, prostate, sciatica, leg, knee, and foot problems.

2ⁿᵈ Center:
Located in the abdominal region of the body, this center is associated with emotions, relationships, creativity, finances, and sexuality. This center is about relationships of all kinds.

Energetic Drains: Negative emotional addictions. Fear over finances. Lack of relationship skills.

Archetypes:
Unhealthy Expression: The Abused Child
Healthy Expression: The Creative Goddess/God

Diseases Associated with The 2ⁿᵈ Center:
Bowel diseases (IBS, Crohn's, leaky gut, colon cancer), diseases of the genitals (endometriosis, cancer of the prostate, testicles, ovaries, cervix), lower back problems.

3rd Center:

Located in the area of the stomach, also known as the solar plexus, this center has to do with personal power, confidence, intuition (gut feelings/hunches). This center is about your confidence and feelings of power in your own life and with others around you.

Energetic Drains: Eroded sense of self, self-deprecation, self-loathing, and self-hatred. Controlling self and others.

Archetypes:

Unhealthy Expression: The Slacker
Healthy Expression: The Successful CEO

Diseases associated with the 3rd center:

Ulcers, stomach cancers, kidney diseases, gallbladder disease, liver diseases.

4th Center:

Located in the area of the heart, this center is all about universal love, forgiveness, compassion, and truth. This center is the balancing agent between the lower centers associated with earthly life and the upper centers associated with your spiritual/energetic life. It is about higher, unconditional love.

Archetypes:

Unhealthy Expression: The Victim
Healthiest Expression: The Lover of All

Diseases associated with the 4th center:

Heart disease, lung diseases (COPD, lung cancer), thymus gland issues, upper back & shoulder pain and problems.

5th Center:

Located in the area of the throat, this center is about communication, expression, choice, and higher will. This center is about your personal expression and living up to the full potential of who you are meant to be on this Earth. You use your power of choice to create and communicate your mission and purpose using this center.

Archetypes:
Unhealthy Expression: The Drama King/Queen
Healthiest Expression: The Wise Sage

Diseases associated with the 5th Center:
All thyroid diseases, esophageal cancers, neck problems, chronic laryngitis and throat clearing.

6th Center:

Located in the area of the forehead, this center has long been associated with the mystical and unexplainable attributes of clairvoyance (seeing beyond the physical), clairaudience (hearing beyond the physical), clairsentience (the sense of knowing something without physical evidence). It is the mind's eye, also known as the third eye and sometimes referred to as the "mental field".

Archetypes:
Unhealthiest form: The Stepford Wife
Healthiest form: The Enlightened Yogi

Diseases associated with the 6ᵗʰ center:
Brain disorders, brain tumors, migraines, eye diseases, hearing loss, chronic ear infections.

7ᵗʰ Center:
Located at the top of the head, this is the spiritual center connected to the Universe, God, or however you see the higher power. It is associated with your personal connection to the spiritual/energetic. In near death experiences, there are numerous documented cases of people saying it felt like they "popped out of the top of their heads" when they briefly died, and "popped back into their bodies" at the top of the head when they came back to life.

Archetypes:
Unhealthiest form: The Curmudgeon
Healthiest form: The Avatar/Guru

Diseases associated with the 7ᵗʰ Center:
Alcoholism, drug addiction, sex addiction, food addiction – addictions of all kinds are a spiritual/energetic cry for help.

Archetypes and Their Power
You'll see I have created archetypes for each of the centers of The Human Energy System. An archetype is a collective idea about anything that humans generally understand. For instance, there is an archetype for "teacher". We all know what a teacher is. Within the archetype of teacher, there are sub archetypes that specify the kind of teacher. These would be things like; "Awful Teacher", "Wise Teacher", "The Absent-

Minded Professor". These are all ideas that we can relate to in some way.

I have added archetypes to the various centers of the Human Energy System to help you get an idea of what I've repeatedly seen as healthy and unhealthy ways that people tend to be stuck in a particular energy center and the opposite energy which is how they can resolve that energy center, gaining more energy to run their biological systems.

For instance, say you've got stomach ulcers. You can recognize that your personal power is being drained by holding down a job you absolutely hate, and you're incredibly stressed out, anxious, fearful, and upset every single day that you do this job you despise. When you look at the third center of the Human Energy system and the associated archetypes, you see "The Slacker" and the "CEO".

You may think to yourself that you are anything but a slacker and that all you do is work in a job you hate. And you may get really upset and offended at the notion of being a slacker. What you are slacking on may be that you're not honoring your own inner calling to create the life you desire by working towards something you've always wanted to do, using your skills, talents, and abilities to do that. It may be that you lack the confidence to do the thing you really love or perhaps others around you are the naysayers that keep criticizing your efforts. It is up to you to find the confidence to create the life you desire to live and/or, to change your relationship to your current job so that you can emotionally resolve your issues and thus, your ulcers. Confidence is the emotion that builds this center up to operate as fully functional.

Think of each of the centers of this system and the associated archetypes and see where you may feel you need help. You may enter this door through your disease. So, say you have colon cancer. The colon is in the second center of the Human Energy System. You see that the archetypes are The Wounded Child and

The Creative God/Goddess. Immediately you think of how your parent abused you as a child. This sudden flash of insight is the very thing that may be the root cause of the disease and only you can set that abused child free with the help of a great guide. That will come from realizing yourself as a creative God/Goddess.

The idea of going from wounded child to God seems daunting and impossible. Just take one step at a time. Look at the God archetype – all love, all the time. What is one thing you can do right now to show the wounded child within you that you love him or her? Perhaps you can do a simple meditation, visualizing a God or Goddess holding and healing your wounded child. Perhaps you can take yourself out for a movie or something that makes your child-self feel loved and cared for. The unconscious mind communicates in symbols and archetypes – the child is an archetype that often holds the keys to your own healing and forward movement.

You have many, many aspects of you operating simultaneously. Which one will you develop to come to the forefront? Which aspect will you give the most love and attention to? You have the power to create your illness unconsciously. How about creating health and wellness in your body consciously? Why not at least set out to heal what could possibly be at the root of why you got sick in the first place?

Archetypes can be useful tools for you to achieve healing. You never know what will be the thing that can turn your illness around. I have seen clients turn it around with one thought that led to a deep sense of self understanding. Keep your mind and heart open to the possibility that you're getting well is just one thought away.

When I was first introduced to this way of thinking, I was seriously skeptical. I thought it was all conjecture and, even though it made sense, it didn't seem like it could make me well. I was raised by a scientist and a defense contractor; two logical parents who trained me to think logically. What did I do? I chose to open my mind to a marriage between ancient wisdom and modern-day science and to combine the two. I still approach new and out there ideas with skepticism – I think that is healthy to question, investigate, and open your mind to new possibilities.

If it doesn't work for me, I move on. I encourage you to do the same. There are infinite ways to get well. Keep moving towards your healing and everything you need will be provided for you.

10

A PLAN FOR CHANGE

Through the decades of my personal healing, the study of it, and working with hundreds of clients, I have found many tools that can help you on your pathway to get well and stay that way. The most important one, I would have to say is creating a plan for your change. From creating a food plan with shopping lists to a therapy plan for healing underlying contributing factors to your illness, making some sort of concrete statement of what you would like to accomplish and how you would like to get there is incredibly beneficial.

There is something powerful about stating what you want and finding the people that will help you get that. If getting well is what you want, finding a team of healers to help you is necessary as you cannot do it alone. I tried to read the books and follow that advice way back when, but the true healing came when I sought the help that I needed and the practitioners that could assist me in my goals.

That fateful moment while reading the article on alternative medicine in Washingtonian Magazine back in 1995 led me to seek chiropractic care for the issues associated with scoliosis and a ruptured disc in my neck. That doctor suggested a nutritionist, a yoga instructor, and a massage therapist to add to my team of healers. As I rapidly felt so much better for the first time since I could remember, I became obsessed with alternative methods and tried everything I could get my hands that felt right to try.

You may be thinking about how expensive that all got. It came out of my own pocket because insurance did not cover any of my care outside of western medical practices. I was having such rapid relief that I did not care how much it cost – and I certainly didn't have much money as I was only making $25,000.00 a year. Somehow, the money always came for exactly what I needed, and I got well. As long as I stayed in the western allopathic care system, I got sicker and more dependent on the drugs they prescribed that only masked symptoms and create side effects. If I could figure out how to get well using my diet and alternative care, to me, that was priceless, and I have always found a way to do it. I know you can too.

Where to Start

There are so many choices for alternative care these days it is astounding. Back when I started, there were very few people seeking these methods and most people truly thought that people who went to alternative practitioners were crazy. While it is far more accepted now, there is still a chasm between the alternative and the allopathic communities that is quite deep. The fact remains that western, allopathic medicine is only a couple hundred years old and traditional medicinal methods have been saving humanity for thousands of years. There are merits to both fields and doctors that combine both are the ones I tend to recommend. I shy away from elitism in any field. Meaning, that sense that they are the one and only solution for you to better your life and get well. That thinking can be potentially dangerous.

Today, there is movement towards something called Functional Medicine. It is based in searching for and treating the root cause of illness using food, supplements, exercise, and western medicine combined. It is such a new field of study and there is so much to be learned by the western medical physicians that use functional medical practices that I would still highly recommend combining various treatments like acupuncture, herbal medicine, spiritual psychotherapy, reiki, and/or chiropractic care to create a comprehensive healing plan for you.

Suggested Healing Modalities

There are so many different healing modalities you can use to create your wellness plan. I have come across SO many over the years that putting together a list will not likely do justice to all the potential methods that are out there.

I have listed some of the more popular ones and a brief description of them. See what resonates with you and consider using practitioners in these modalities to help you.

Chiropractic Care

Acupuncture

Rolfing

Transpersonal Psychotherapy – Ro-Hun, Inner Child Therapy

Past life regression therapy

Reiki/The Radiance Technique

Healing Touch

Cranial Sacral Therapy

Shamanic Healing

Chinese Herbal Medicine

QXCI Healing Machines

Homeopathy

Meditation

Yoga

Hypnotherapy

Emotional Freedom Technique

Whole Person Integration Technique

These therapies listed begin the scratch the surface of what is out there to use as healing modalities for your wellness. Look into them to see what feels right for you. One interesting way that I determine which way to go lies in the intuitive for me. If I hear the same modality suggested to me three times or more in a small space of time, I explore it.

Remember I said that when you make a decision to get well that everything you need just starts to show up for you? It's truly miraculous but it does. People, opportunities, modalities, books, films, and everything you need just begins to come to you. Not everything you try may give you the results you want. In some cases you may need to stick with things for a while, in others, you may need to move on if you feel that the modality you're trying isn't making any difference.

You will learn to trust the process and, more importantly, trust yourself. You've got the answers inside of you to your own healing. You've got this. I have faith in you.

11

CREATING A NEW WAY OF THOUGHT

I n my experience, it is mindset that is at the very core of your wellness journey. Without that, it is a rare event that you will get well. There are miracles that happen, yes, but I have rarely seen them happen without some sort of action made along the way that included determination, passion, planning, intuition, prayer, intention, decision, and a deep desire to get well, both on the part of the person who is sick and the people around them.

Isabel's Story

She's my sister soul mate, "my bestest friend in the whole wide world", as we have been telling one another since we were small children. She's also the mother of the three kids God gave me to help raise. Especially after her heart stopped.

We were 38 years old. It was 5:30 on a May morning in 2006, when the seizure began. She lost oxygen to her brain for at least ten minutes until the paramedics came to revive her. The defribulators were used the maximum number of times allowed. On the last shock, they brought her back.

She was rushed to the emergency room where she flailed on a gurney for the next nine hours until they induced a coma, so she could rest. They told us that she would likely not live and if she did, she would be a vegetable for the rest of her life.

I could feel her spirit standing beside me in the ER, with her husband and children gathered around her. She communicated that we should not let go. I know it sounds fantastical and impossible, but I experienced her with me. I turned to all the family and said; "She's going to make it. We are not giving up on her. We all need to be united in believing she will come back to us. No other option is acceptable." We all agreed with great conviction that she would heal.

I spent the next two and a half months at her ICU bedside, sending healing light and love with Authentic Reiki (Radiance Technique), a hands-on healing technique that produces healing by working with the human energy system. We brought in the priest from their Episcopal Church to anoint her with oils as close friends gathered at her bedside in prayer with focused intention to help her get well. We put her on prayer lists all over the world in both religious and spiritual traditions, pulling out all the stops for anything that could help her recover.

Her organ systems shut down one by one. It was as if each organ had to re-boot and start up again. On the night her kidneys shut down, they called the family in and told us she would not likely make it through the night. We still held tight to her healing. Her then husband and I spent that entire night with her. I held one hand and he held the other, sending prayers and love to her all-night long.

One month earlier after she went into the hospital, I had put a call into my friends at Delphi University, requesting vibhutti (sacred ash) from Sai Baba, a saint in India who could create healing miracles with this ash that smelled like roses. They told me they turned the place upside down and could not find it anywhere.

On the day that Isabel's kidneys shut down, I received a call from Delphi. A vial of this healing ash appeared on the desk of the president of the University. They remembered my request and called me to ask if I still needed it. I did. Isabel needed it more than ever. They sent it overnight and I used it on her hands, feet, and on her tongue as instructed. She came back to us that day and spent the next four months recovering, learning to walk, talk, eat, write, draw, and communicate with us all over again.

Isabel is still with us 12 years later. She is termed "severely brain damaged" but she can do so much. She can cook, write, care for herself, create, share ideas, and carry on great conversations. Her memory is not good. Her ability for higher reasoning is not nearly what it once was. She can't drive, but she is high functioning for what happened to her and able to spend time with her children and grandson who thinks she is just the greatest person ever. She is. She is a miracle.

Do you see how this miracle was a participatory event? We all took action. We all focused our intentions for her wellness and prayed for the best possible outcome for our dear Isabel. We had hundreds of people all over the world praying for her. I kept a daily blog of what was happening with her to communicate to loved ones everywhere and to help me keep my sanity because it was a harrowing experience.

There was someone by her side every moment. I made up a schedule where family, friends, and church parishioners could sit with Isabel, reading to her, singing to her, massaging her hands and feet so she could know she was never, ever alone. Her kids were there every day talking to her, sharing their updates with her although she was unable to understand what they were saying. We just kept loving her.

Miracles do happen. They are more likely to happen when we band together with others to create them. Miracles are an act of creation and we are all capable of producing them. We all have what we need inside of ourselves to heal and assist others. It's not hocus pocus. It's not cryptic. It all starts with a decision.

The action of deciding on a miracle is the best decision you will ever make. Be ready for anything because sometimes your miracle will come a long way down the pike. It rarely ever happens the way you expect it to. Often it turns out much better than you could have ever imagined. Just be open to receiving what the brilliance of the energy of miracles has to provide for you. Expect them and they will come. Accept the package it comes in and you will create happiness for you and those around you.

The Most Important Thought

If there is one thing I can impart to you it's this: *your healing is up to you* and those around you when you cannot be present to be there, like Isabel. You aren't required to believe your doctors. Don't let them tell you that your only option is their prediction. They may be correct, but do you want to prove them right when you are told you have a few months to live? Say no to that. They don't have all the answers. You do.

I met a woman recently who was delivered a catastrophic diagnosis. She was in for a long, slow, painful death according to her doctor. She was devastated. She called her mom to fly in to take care of her child, so she could grieve this loss. The only problem was the diagnosis her doctor gave was an impossible one for her. It was something that only happened to sixty plus year old men – not thirty-six year old women. *She did not have that disease!*

Do not take a diagnosis or a prognosis as the only possible outcome. I have personally witnessed tumors disappear or shrink, I've read of advanced end stage malignant brain tumors going into complete remission. I have heard stories of people who have healed the rarest forms of cancer and disease. I have healed chronic diseases in my own body that I was told would never go away.

Each time I received a new diagnosis, especially the one for Mixed Connective Tissue Disease, I researched what Western Medicine said, mourned the possibility of a long slow death as promised by the western medical profession then I searched around to find someone who had and healed the condition that I had. Each time I did this, I had to re-adopt the mindset necessary to overcome what I had. It's the one where I use my propensity towards stubbornness for my own good. Be stubborn enough to not accept the nasty fate the doctor's hand to you. And always remember that miracles require participation that start with making up your mind that they are expected.

This is your new way of thought. Adopt this determination for wellness and you will be so surprised at all the things and people that show up for you to help you get well. You will witness so many things coming to you that you never dreamed were possible when you awaken to this idea of your healing being in *your own hands*, you are asking for all the people and all of the situations to magnetize to you that will best allow you to get well now.

EPILOGUE

Healing is the process of getting well. Like disease, it does not happen overnight. In order to heal, it takes time, commitment, desire, dedication, and love. It takes the engagement of your entire holistic system from your mind, emotions, physical body, and energetic body. True and lasting healing is a holistic process that involves the different parts of you.

There is never one moment of your life in which you are not engaging the whole of you to do anything. Your heart is always beating, your lungs are always breathing, your mind is always thinking, and your emotions are always emoting, whether you are aware of those processes or not. All these things are working in tandem for your greater good or towards your ultimate destruction.

Yes, we will all die someday, but you have so much more say in how that happens than you can possibly understand. You have the great gift of will power and choice and the free will to use them to evolve and heal.

In the US today people are dying as many as 75 years earlier than they probably should. One woman told me that her friend would justify her terrible food choices and lifestyle by saying; "I don't care if I die one month earlier than I probably should because I eat junk food." Meh. One month. Who really cares, right? The thing is, that is not what is happening. People are leaving the planet in droves in industrialized nations like the U.S. ten, twenty, thirty, fifty years earlier than they should.

We are led to believe that we are living so much longer now because of all the advancements in western medicine. That may be true to some extent – they do incredible things now! They have also handled infectious diseases quite well that used to take out huge portions of the population. I just see so many people living on multiple medicines, uncomfortable procedures, multiple surgeries, and machinery that is keeping them alive and sick for decades. *Alive and sick.* Not alive and well and living life fully. I don't know about you, but I want to be alive and well and really living. But with the trajectory that I was on nearly twenty-five years ago, I was sick and getting sicker. That is what this book is birthed from – that place of seeking wellness instead of long term, chronic, *never going to go away* illness.

If you have read to these last words, I commend you for your dedication to your own health and wellness. You are an incredibly special person and I absolutely adore you! Your contribution to your own health, along with your willingness to take your healing into your own hands will change the world. What you do for you is done for the greater good of all.

Right before my mom and I hang up the phone she always says; "Take good care of my baby." I always say back, with complete confidence; "I will!"

Take good care of your mama's baby. There is only one you. You are precious, and we need your skills, talents, abilities, and love to make this world a more empowered place.

Thank you! I love you!

Dr. Meg Haworth
  March 22, 2018
  Hollywood, California

ABOUT THE AUTHOR

Born in Washington DC to a scientist mother and a defense contractor father, Meg Haworth came into the world as a gentle, sweet, creative, sensitive soul with an introverted and shy disposition. She was born at the height of the summer of love in 1967 but could not have been any further from the energy of open, explorative, creative, artful consciousness that permeated the movement of free love and self-expression. Her strict, religious, rule filled upbringing – coupled with trauma – created the exact dissonance she would need to eventually become a pioneer in holistic health, wellness, healthy cooking, and the pioneering field of Transpersonal Psychology.

At an early age, she had an uncanny ability to know what people were thinking, feeling, and hiding. She spent years honing these natural gifts to assist herself in her personal evolution and then help others. She uses her intuitive skills to help clients transcend their deepest wounds and overcome their mental, emotional, physical and energetic disparities.

Dr. Meg Haworth has spent over two decades in the arena of health, nutrition, and holistic medicine, owning a bed & breakfast and retreat center, conducting workshops, leading numerous wild dolphin retreats in the Bahamas, working with hundreds of clients, speaking, teaching workshops, overseeing a hospital speaker's program, teaching cooking classes, developing recipes, publishing numerous articles, writing six books, co-authoring two additional books, hosting a radio show and a podcast series, teaching cooking classes at Whole Foods and Earth Fare Natural

Foods Markets, producing over fifty cooking videos, being featured on NBC Nightly News, The LA Times and the Huffington Post, and being interviewed on numerous expert summits and online master classes. Dr. Meg's obsession is with health, wellness and communicating that to the masses so they too, can heal themselves.

She lives in Hollywood, California with her sweet dog Diego.

Get Well Now Programs

Dr. Meg Haworth offers a number of programs to assist people with holistic wellness. She focuses mainly on women who were sexually, physically, or emotionally abused as children and now have a chronic illness. She uses the ACE Quiz from the Adverse Childhood Experiences Study – linking childhood abuse and family dysfunction with chronic illnesses later in life – to asses her clients need and get them pointed in the direction that will best suit their needs.

Along with the ACE Quiz (a simple ten question quiz), she offers her free e-book *10 Steps to Overcoming the Effects of Victimization* which contains her Whole Person Integration Technique – a method that works with processing stuck emotions in the body and releasing them at the cellular level. She also offers a free anti-inflammatory lunch recipe for people on the go cook book. To get this trifecta of gifts, go to www.meghaworth.com

Also, on her home page, you can sign up for a free twenty-minute phone or internet consultation to assess your ACE Quiz score and talk about what steps to take next on your own healing pathway. Dr. Meg stresses that even if you ACE score is a 1, you may have significant fallout from that one category. Do not let your score deter you from speaking with her for free if you feel led to talk with her.

Dr. Meg offers an online course to learn the fundamentals of eating foods that heal the body and support it to heal itself while the inner work is happening. To get *21 Days to Healthy Eating,* complete with 21 easy recipes (all created for her celebrity chef clients), resources, teachings, and bonus cooking videos, go to www.meghaworth.com/shop

To have a food plan tailored to your specific needs to support healing a specific condition you may have, you can work with Dr. Meg directly in her program *What Celebrities Eat*, where you get the same star treatment her celebrity clients get as a private chef in Hollywood. You will have a food plan, recipes created just for you, personal recommendations, and specific instruction on how to carry out your plan directly with her.

For a more comprehensive program that covers your personalized food plan, an environmental assessment, and the inner Transpersonal work necessary to truly heal, Dr. Meg offers her program, *Get Well Now*, a three month one on one program to help you heal your chronic illness on all levels. The program takes you through a holistic process, mapping out an individual plan created specifically for you. She covers your diet, environment, and inner emotional life for a full transformational package to wellness.

Many clients opt for one on one sessions over the phone, Skype, FaceTime, Facebook Messenger, or WhatsApp for individualized work that helps them heal one session at a time. Those sessions are available in multi session package rates.

Dr. Meg has two online Facebook groups for health and wellness:

Get Well Now; IBS Fibromyalgia & Chronic Illness Support Group and *Lightning Women; Healing the wounds of childhood sexual, physical and emotional abuse* – for women only to talk about their histories of abuse and to have a place to be inspired to overcome our wounds together.

Available on iTunes and Sound Cloud, is Dr. Meg's Podcast series, *Get Well with Dr. Meg Haworth*, in which she interviews the top wellness experts on the planet today, bringing you the current science and innovations in health and wellness with luminaries like JJ Virgin on Traumatic Brain Injuries, Dr. Steven Masley on better solutions for brain health, Chris Wark from Chris Beat Cancer on what every cancer patient needs to know, Dr. Eric Zielinski on the healing power of essential oils, Wynn Claybaugh, owner of the Paul Mitchell Salon Schools on the healing power of being nice, Joe Cross, from the documentaries, *Fat Sick & Nearly Dead I & II* on whether or not juicing is right for you and so many more and Dr. David Friedman on bringing sanity back to your food choices. You can find all of the podcasts on my blog at www.meghaworth.com/blog or at the iTunes store when you search for *Get Well Soon*.

To get a copy of my book and guide for going gluten and dairy free, *Done with Dairy. Giving up Gluten; 14 Days to a Delicious and Healthy You*, go to www.meghaworth.com/shop

To receive Dr. Meg's weekly newsletter, go to her website to sign up at www.meghaworth.com – You will also receive the *ACE Quiz, 10 Steps to Overcoming the Effects of Victimization* and *5 Anti-Inflammatory Lunch Recipes for People on the Go.*

You can follow Dr. Meg on all social media platforms @drmeghaworth and/or @thelightningwomen on Instagram, Twitter and Linkedin. On Facebook by searching Meg Haworth or on her fan page www.facebook.com/coachdrmeghaworth or on her group pages (as listed above). *Lightning Women* is a secret group, so you will have to ask her directly to join via e-mail or messaging.

To email her directly, you can go to meg@meghaworth.com

Her web address is www.meghaworth.com

REFERENCES

Natural Resources Defense Council. (2018) Home Page "Of the more than 80,000 Chemicals. Retrieved from https://www.nrdc.org/issues/toxic-chemicals

U.S. Food and Drug Administration. (2011 April). Guidance for Industry: Questions and Answers About the Petition Process. [Web Page] https://www.fda.gov/Food/GuidanceRegulation/GuidanceDocumentsRegulatoryInformation/ucm253328.htm

American Heart Association. (2018). Trans Fats. [Blog Post] http://www.heart.org/HEARTORG/HealthyLiving/FatsAnd-Oils/Fats101/Trans-Fats_UCM_301120_Article.jsp#.W2ZVAihKhPY

Yale Journal of Biology and Medicine. (2010 June). Gain weight by "going diet?" Artificial sweeteners and the neurobiology of sugar cravings. [Article] https://www.ncbi.nlm.nih.gov/pmc/articles/PMC2892765/

Mercola. (2015 March 18). Study Links Common Food Additives to Crohn's Disease, Colitis. [Blog Post] https://articles.mercola.com/sites/articles/archive/2015/03/18/food-additives-crohns-disease-colitis.aspx

Harvard T.H. Chan School of Public Health. (2015 November

3). WHO report says eating processed meat is carcinogenic: Understanding the findings. [Web Page] https://www.hsph.harvard.edu/nutritionsource/2015/11/03/report-says-eating-processed-meat-is-carcinogenic-understanding-the-findings/

National Institute of Environmental Health Sciences. (2010 October). Diet and Nutrition: The Artificial Food Dye Blues. [Journal   Article] https://www.ncbi.nlm.nih.gov/pmc/articles/PMC2957945/

Scientific American. (2015 March 25). Widely Used Herbicide Linked to Cancer. [Blog Post] https://www.scientificamerican.com/article/widely-used-herbicide-linked-to-cancer/

US National Library of Medicine National Institutes of Health. (1994 Fall). Excitotoxins in foods. [Article] https://www.ncbi.nlm.nih.gov/pubmed/7854587

Dr. Mercola. (2014 July 4). MSG: What This "Delicious" Ingredient Can Do to Your Health. http://www.drmercola.com/obesity/msg-what-this-delicious-ingredient-can-do-to-your-health/

Pesticide Action Network International. (2018 April 30). Consolidated List of Banned Pesticides. http://pan-international.org/pan-international-consolidated-list-of-banned-pesticides/

European Food Safety Authority. (2018 August 2). Food Additives. https://www.efsa.europa.eu/en/topics/topic/food-additives

National Center for Biotechnology Information. (2013 May 1). Combined pesticide exposure severely affects individual- and colony- level traits in bees. [Abstract]https://www.ncbi.nlm.nih.gov/pmc/articles/PMC3495159/

Pub Med. U.S. National Library of Medicine National Institutes of Health. (2012 November). Long term toxicity of Roundup herbicide and Roundup tolerant genetically modified maize. [Abstract] https://www.ncbi.nlm.nih.gov/pubmed/22999595

National Institutes of Health News in Health. (2014 February). Stop the Spread of Superbugs; Help Fight Drug-Resistant Bacteria. [Newsletter] https://newsinhealth.nih.gov/2014/02/stop-spread-superbugs

Medical News Today. (2017 August 1). Nine ways that processed foods are harming people. [Newsletter] https://www.medicalnewstoday.com/articles/318630.php

UCLA Newsroom. (2008 July 9). Scientists learn how what you eat affects your brain – and those of your kids. [Blog Post]. http://newsroom.ucla.edu/releases/scientists-learn-how-food-affects-52668

Pub Med. US National Library of Medicine National Institutes of Health. (1997 November 12). Glutamate in neurologic diseases. [Abstract] https://www.ncbi.nlm.nih.gov/pubmed/943031

Centers for Disease Control and Prevention. (2018 July 31). Cancer Data and Statistics. [Web Page] https://www.cdc.gov/cancer/dcpc/data/index.htm

Extoxnet. Toxic Information Brief. Cornell University. (1993 September). Entry and Fate of Chemicals in Humans. [Publication]
http://pmep.cce.cornell.edu/profiles/extoxnet/TIB/entry.html

National Institutes of Environmental Health Sciences; Environmental Health Perspectives. (2016 Volume 124). Parabens and Human Epidermal Growth Factor Receptor Ligand Cross-Talk in Breast Cancer Cells. [Journal Article]. https://ehp.niehs.nih.gov/14-09200/

Environmental Working Group. (2018). Know your Environment. Protect your health. [Website] https://www.ewg.org/

US National Library of Medicine National Institutes of Health. (2016 October 1). Dietary Triggers in Irritable Bowel Syndrome; Is There a Role for Gluten? [Abstract] https://www.ncbi.nlm.nih.gov/pmc/articles/PMC5056565/

National Center for Biotechnology Information. (2011). Herbal Medicine: Biomolecular and Clinical Aspects; 2nd Edition. [Webpage] https://www.ncbi.nlm.nih.gov/books/NBK92773/

Johns Hopkins University HUB. (2016 May 3). Johns Hopkins Study Suggests Medical Errors are Thid-Leading Cause of Death in U.S. [Journal] https://hub.jhu.edu/2016/05/03/medical-errors-third-leading-cause-of-death/

American Cancer Society; Cancer Action Network. (2017 April). The Costs of Cancer; Addressing Patient Costs. [Article] https://www.acscan.org/sites/default/files/Costs%20of%20-Cancer%20-%20Final%20Web.pdf

Oxford Academic Journal of the National Cancer Institute. (1999 August 4). Cancer Risk in BRCA-2 Mutation Carriers. [Article] https://academic.oup.com/jnci/article/91/15/1310/2543764

US National Library of Medicine National Institutes of Health. (2006 March). Epigenetics: The Science of Change. [Article] https://www.ncbi.nlm.nih.gov/pmc/articles/PMC1392256/

UCLA History & Special Collections; Louise M. Darling Biomedical Library. (2002) Medical Uses of Spices. [Webpage] https://unitproj.library.ucla.edu/biomed/spice/index.cfm?spice-filename=medspice.txt&itemsuppress=yes&displayswitch=0

Whole Foods Market. (2018). Quality Standards. [Webpage] https://www.wholefoodsmarket.com/quality-standards

Environmental Health Perspectives. (2016 April 13). Recent Fast Food Consumption and Bisphenol-A and Phthalates Exposure Among the U.S. Populations in NHANES 2003-2010. [Advance Publication] https://ehp.niehs.nih.gov/wp-content/uploads/advpub/2016/4/ehp.1510803.acco.pdf

Davis, William, MD. (2011) Wheat Belly; Lose the Wheat, Lose the Weight and Find Your Path Back to Health. Rodale.

Zukav, Gary (1989) Seat of The Soul. Simon & Schuster. New York, New York.

American Cancer Society. (2018) DES Exposure: Questions an Answers. [Web Page] https://www.cancer.org/cancer/cancer-causes/medical-treatments/des-exposure.html

US National Library of Medicine National Institutes of Health. (2009 Fall). The Risks of Not Breasfeeding for Mothers and Infants. [Article] https://www.cancer.org/cancer/cancer-causes/medical-treatments/des-exposure.html

Centers for Disease Control and Prevention. (2018) Adverse Childhood Experiences Study (ACEs). [Web Page] https://www.cdc.gov/violenceprevention/acestudy/index.html

Myss, Caroline. (1996) Anatomy of The Spirit; The Seven Stages of Power and Healing.Penguin Random House, LLC.

OTHER BOOKS BY DR. MEG HAWORTH, PH.D.

Inspiration to Realization; Volume III (Co-Author)

Become Who You Are; The Stages of Spiritual Transformation –
Workbooks I, II, and III

Audacious Creativity (Co-Author)

Done with Dairy. Giving up Gluten; 14 Days to a Delicious and Healthy
You

Dining Out Without Gluten and Dairy

Made in the USA
Middletown, DE
26 October 2018